HEALTHY LIVING from A to Z

Praise for
HEALTHY LIVING from A to Z

"With an honest and encouraging voice, Rhonda Huff coaches the reader on a wellness journey, addressing emotional, nutritional, physical and cognitive components of a healthy life. All of the tools are here, garnered from the author's years of experience, to lead each of us to develop a thriving body, mind and spirit. Healthy Living from A to Z offers a blueprint for a personalized wellness approach that both my patients and I can use."

—Jennifer McCord, MD, IFMCP,
Co-founder, The Center for Integrative Brain Health

"After reviewing *Healthy Living from A to Z*, I am happily endorsing this professional intuitive book that makes you feel part of each chapter. It is fresh and so simple to follow along that you can't wait for the next chapter. I know this book will help a lot of people explore themselves in a deep dive for ultimate and comprehensive health. Rhonda's suggestions, supported with simple, easy to understand research, are so user friendly that you are excited to take the journey to a healthier you. Congrats Rhonda!!"

—Jay DelVecchio
President & CEO, World Instructor Training Schools

"On our unique healing journey, Rhonda's empowering presentation style provides a profound synthesis of joy, creativity and expertise and gives us renewed enthusiasm for life and wholeness. A delight to read!"

— Sinclair B. McCracken, MD, IFMCP
Founder, Sinclair Health, PC,
Functional Medicine and Bioenergetic Wellness

"This gem of a book is a map to lifelong health using simple, effective and holistic approaches."

—Jack Mantione MSPT, DPT, QNCP, CSCS,
Creator, The Mantione Method
Owner, The Mantione Center for Sports Rehabilitation

HEALTHY
LIVING

from A to Z

*The Guide to Finding Who You
Really Are and Feeding Who
You Were Created to Be*

Rhonda Huff, M.E.d., B.S.

NEW YORK

LONDON • NASHVILLE • MELBOURNE • VANCOUVER

HEALTHY LIVING from A to Z
The Guide to Finding Who You Really Are and Feeding Who You Were Created to Be

© 2019 Rhonda Huff, M.E.d., B.S.

Published in New York, New York, by Morgan James Publishing. Morgan James is a trademark of Morgan James, LLC. www.MorganJamesPublishing.com

ISBN 978-1-64279-314-7 paperback
ISBN 978-1-64279-315-4 eBook
Library of Congress Control Number: 2018912158

Cover Design by:
Rachel Lopez
www.r2cdesign.com

Interior Design by:
Bonnie Bushman
The Whole Caboodle Graphic Design

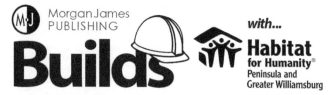

In an effort to support local communities, raise awareness and funds, Morgan James Publishing donates a percentage of all book sales for the life of each book to Habitat for Humanity Peninsula and Greater Williamsburg.

Get involved today! Visit
www.MorganJamesBuilds.com

DEDICATION

To everyone who wakes up and chooses
to rise above their circumstances.

TABLE OF CONTENTS

Foreword   xiii

Preface   xv

    What Does it Mean to be Healthy?   *xv*

Acknowledgements   xix

Introduction   xx

Chapter A Prep   1

Chapter A   3

    Emotional Health: Affirmations   *3*

    Nutritional Health: Add More Green   *4*

    Physical Health: Active Release/Trigger Point Therapy/Self Myofascial Release   *6*

    Cognitive Health: ABC...ZYX   *7*

Chapter B Prep   8

Chapter B   9

    Emotional Health: Breathe   *9*

    Nutritional Health: Build a Better Plan   *10*

    Physical Health: Bedtime   *12*

    Cognitive Health: Brain Food   *16*

Chapter C Prep   21

Chapter C   22

    Emotional Health: Circle of Life   *22*

    Nutritional Health: Cravings   *24*

    Physical Health: Corrective Exercise   *26*

    Cognitive Health: Crosswords   *28*

Chapter D Prep   30

Chapter D   31

    Emotional Health: Distress or Eustress?   *31*

    Nutritional Health: Disordered Eating   *34*

    Physical Health: Dosha and Exercise   *38*

    Cognitive Health: Dance   *42*

Chapter E Prep   44

Chapter E   46

    Emotional Health: Emotional Tune-up   *46*

    Nutritional Health: Eliminations   *48*

    Physical Health: Exercise   *50*

    Cognitive Health: Evaluating Core Beliefs   *53*

Chapter F Prep   57

Chapter F   59

    Emotional Health: Four Agreements   *59*

    Nutritional Health: FOOD©   *61*

    Physical Health: Floss and Scrape   *65*

    Fifteen Fun Facts About Your Brain   *66*

Chapter G Prep   68

Chapter G   70

    Emotional Health: Grief's Positive Purpose—the Goodbye Exercise   *70*

    Nutritional Health: Gut Health   *72*

    Physical Health: Glutes   *75*

    Cognitive Health: Gratitude   *76*

Chapter H Prep   78

Chapter H   81

    Emotional Health: Highly Sensitive People   *81*

    Nutritional Health: Hot or Cold?   *82*

    Physical Health: Heat It Up   *84*

    Cognitive Health: Hypnosis   *88*

Chapter I Prep   90

Chapter I   92

    Emotional Health: Ideal Worksheet   *92*

Nutritional Health: Intermittent Fasting *93*

Physical Health: Interval Training *94*

Cognitive Health: Intuition *101*

Chapter J Prep 105

Chapter J 107

 Emotional Health: Journaling *107*

 Nutritional Health: Juicing *109*

 Physical Health: Joints *111*

 Cognitive Health: Juggling *112*

Chapter K Prep 114

Chapter K 116

 Emotional Health: Kindness *116*

 Nutritional Health: Kitchen Cleanup *117*

 Physical Health: Kyphosis *121*

 Cognitive Health: Kryptonite for the Brain *122*

Chapter L Prep 124

Chapter L 126

 Emotional Health: Love Languages *126*

 Nutritional Health: Leaky Gut Syndrome *128*

 Physical Health: Laughter *129*

 Cognitive Health: Learn Something New *130*

Chapter M Prep 131

Chapter M 133

 Emotional Health: Myers-Briggs Personality Test *133*

 Nutritional Health: Macro-nutrients and Micro-nutrients *134*

 Physical Health: Make-up and Skincare *137*

 Cognitive Health: Map It! *139*

Chapter N Prep 140

Chapter N 142

 Emotional Health: Negativity *142*

 Nutritional Health: Nutritional Deficiencies *143*

 Physical Health: No Equipment Required *145*

 Cognitive Health: Nondominance Exercise *145*

Chapter O Prep   146
Chapter O   148
    Emotional Health: Owning Up   *148*
    Nutritional Health: Orange   *150*
    Physical Health: Outdoor Activities   *150*
    Cognitive Health: Occupational Inventory   *151*

Chapter P Prep   153
Chapter P   154
    Emotional Health: Peacefulness   *154*
    Nutritional Health: Psychology of Food   *155*
    Physical Health: Pain Management   *156*
    Cognitive Health: Poetry   *158*

Chapter Q Prep   160
Chapter Q   161
    Emotional Health: Quiet Time   *161*
    Nutritional Health: Quarter Your Plate   *162*
    Physical Health: Quality over Quantity   *162*
    Cognitive Health: Question Everything   *163*

Chapter R Prep   164
Chapter R   165
    Emotional Health: Responding Instead of Reacting *165*
    Nutritional Health: Red/Purple/Blue/Black   *166*
    Physical Health: Rest and Recovery   *166*
    Cognitive Health: Rules of Brain Health   *168*

Chapter S Prep   170
Chapter S   171
    Emotional Health: Setting Healthy Boundaries *171*
    Nutritional Health: Superfoods   *173*
    Physical Health: Sets and Reps   *174*
    Cognitive Health: Sudoku   *176*

Chapter T Prep   177
Chapter T   178
    Emotional Health: Thought-provoking Questions *178*

Nutritional Health: Taste Your Food *181*

Physical Health: Total Body Workouts *184*

Cognitive Health: Teasers *186*

Chapter U Prep 188

Chapter U 190

Emotional Health: Unmasked *190*

Nutritional Health: Understanding Food Labels *193*

Physical Health: Unilateral Training *194*

Cognitive Health: Unraveling Cognitive Decline…Prevention is KEY *195*

Chapter V Prep 197

Chapter V 199

Emotional Health: Vocalizing the Song Within *199*

Nutritional Health: Vitamins *200*

Physical Health: VO2 Max *210*

Cognitive Health: Vibrations *211*

Chapter W Prep 213

Chapter W 214

Emotional Health: Weaknesses are Strengths Misused *214*

Nutritional Health: Water *215*

Physical Health: Weight Training *216*

Cognitive Health: Wrinkles *217*

Chapter X Prep 218

Chapter X 219

Emotional Health: Xeroxing Life *219*

Nutritional Health: Xenoestrogens *220*

Physical Health: X-traordinary Health *223*

Cognitive Health: Xylophone *224*

Chapter Y Prep 225

Chapter Y 226

Emotional Health: Yes, And! *226*

Nutritional Health: Your Personal Nutrition Plan *227*

Physical Health: Yoga *228*

Cognitive Health: Yawning *229*

Chapter Z Prep   231
Chapter Z   233
    Emotional Health: Zero In On Your Emotional Health   *233*
    Nutritional Health: Zero In On Your Nutritional Health   *235*
    Physical Health: Zero In On Your Physical Health   *237*
    Cognitive Health: Zero In On Your Cognitive Health   *238*
Celebrate the New Healthier YOU   241

About the Author   243
References   244

FOREWORD

I first met Rhonda Huff after reading about her in the newspaper. My neighbor saw me out in the yard and ran over to show me the clip she had saved with the story about Rhonda working with a woman from her church who had multiple sclerosis. The accompanying photo showed the woman with MS on a treadmill.

"I thought maybe she could help YOU," my neighbor said.

The next day at work, the reporter who had written the story came to me asking if I had seen the piece.

"You may want to check her out," the reporter said.

I had to agree. When two people come to you and tell you to do something, you need to do something.

I called Rhonda that day and made an appointment, explaining that I am dealing with a genetic neuromuscular disease known as CMT and had a lifetime fear of treadmills.

It wasn't long before I was on that treadmill and knew that Rhonda was someone special. Not only did she have a wealth of knowledge about health and fitness, she had an intuitive sense about what a person needed and just how much to push them to achieve more. And she had an easy way of communicating that made her knowledge accessible to anyone.

Yes, she worked with people who had disabilities, but she also worked with elite athletes and trained other trainers on ways to motivate their clients to get the best results they had ever seen in their lives.

I saw what she was doing and knew she had to do more to share her message with a broader audience. After dipping her toe into the world of publishing with *The Addictive Personal Trainer*, she has written a guidebook for the masses. With *Healthy Living from A to Z*, Rhonda has created an easy blueprint for anyone to follow that will bring health and healing to everyone in mind, body and spirit.

Many writers tackle the various aspects of wellness in their books on fitness or their promotion of the next diet craze, but few do what Rhonda has done here. To be truly living your best life, you must look at your whole self. She helps us do that here and walks us through the steps to becoming our best, our happiest selves.

—**Karen Turpin Morgan**, Editor

PREFACE

What Does it Mean to be Healthy?

In 1948, the World Health Organization (WHO) defined health as "a state of complete physical, mental and social well-being and not merely the absence of disease or infirmity." Since 1948 the definition has been tweaked a bit and other phrases have been added such as "health is a resource for everyday life," "health is the ability of a body to adapt to new threats and infirmities," and "health is a slippery concept."

If you are like many of the people I coach, you are probably feeling a bit more like health is a slippery concept. After all, every single person on the planet seems to define it differently and every expert has his or her own opinion of the matter.

So why should my opinion matter? Well, I suppose you could say it doesn't. I will be the first one to say that my "opinion" about health has shifted more than a few times over the years. When I was young and in perfect health, my opinion about health was that if someone wasn't healthy then maybe they were just lazy. Then when I was young but not as healthy as discovered through a lupus diagnosis, my opinion became one of complacency and of allowing life to happen to me instead of being an active participant in the process. Over several years that mindset became complete and utter frustration with how no one seemed to have any answers about my health or why was I living in pain all the time. Now I have to tell you, I started working in the fitness field when I was 19 years old and I was 27 at the time of this diagnosis, so even on the days that I didn't feel my best, there were people in my life for whom I had to put on my happy face and push through.

The tipping point finally came after a day and a half of being paralyzed from the waist down and being told "we have no idea what is happening. It must be stress. Just take some time to relax," I decided that life was too long to be sick all the time and I had to do something. I turned to a friend who had been trying to get me to see a Naturopathic Doctor in the area. At the time I honestly thought this was some type of demonic thing, but I had become so desperate to feel better that I agreed to gave it a try. I left that appointment with almost $500 worth of supplements and an attitude that would have made the demons themselves run for cover. But my attitude began changing when after 2 weeks I was feeling better than I had in years and then after 4 weeks I was off every prescription medication and was continuing to feel healthier, stronger, and more energetic.

For about 6 years things were going well and my opinion about health had shifted to more of a follow the food guide pyramid, take some supplements, drink enough water and you will be fine type of philosophy. Then in 2006 I was diagnosed with breast cancer. I looked like the picture of health. I exercised. I ate "right." I worked hard and played hard. But I was still sick. When the doctor gave me the diagnosis my response was, "Well bring me some French fries and ice cream then because apparently it doesn't matter what I eat." He said he had never gotten that reaction before. And we all laughed. But then he immediately began telling me what I needed to do about the cancer. Well, if you have ever had breast cancer, do you remember how hearing words like mastectomy, radiation, and chemotherapy made you feel? Even typing the words right now elicits a feeling that I may throw up. So I naively looked at him and said, "What if I choose to do nothing?" And recalling his response still makes my knees weak, "Then you will die."

If you ask anyone who knows me personally to define me in 3 words or less, I am certain the word "stubborn" would be on every list. And just because I was hearing a cancer diagnosis didn't change that. I decided that I would do my own research, interview some doctors (a bunch of doctors), and get back to him. And I did just that. I said no to the mastectomy, I said no to the radiation, but I did agree to the chemotherapy. They had made a good case about being in and out of the tumor enough times through the biopsies and a lumpectomy to have possibly spread it themselves.

I began chemo with the best attitude in the world! I had on my pink war paint and my Ford "Warriors in Pink" shirt, complete with angel wings, and brought lots of popsicles to share with others who were getting treatments as well. I walked in and offered each person a popsicle but no one accepted. As I walked toward my chair I heard someone say, "it must be her first time." I felt sad but not defeated so I sat there and enjoyed my popsicle in silence. Eventually one lady decided she would take me up on the offer and after that, everyone else did too. Mission accomplished! This drab, horrible place was now filled with people talking to each other and licking on their popsicles. I left feeling like I was healing not only myself but those around me as well. These people were now my people.

I had no idea when I left the clinic that day that my body was about to turn against me in every way possible. Before I could get home, I was on the side of the road hurling my guts out. It was the most horrible feeling of doom that I had ever had. But it had to get better, right? I mean, what body wouldn't rebel against all those toxic chemicals being dripped into it?

The next morning I had to go to work. Now, one year before this happened, I opened a new business. I needed to be able to work while my kids were in school so I did that by opening my own personal training studio where I could work 8-3. No one else worked with me so no one else could work for me. My business wasn't yet strong enough for me to be able to take time off. I had no choice, sick or not, off to work I would go. I have to give some love here. My clients were so supportive of me that they decided that when they came in, they would warm up for 10 minutes on their own so I could lie down. Then they would train with me for the next 50 minutes. The next person would come in, point to the stretching table, and I would obediently and very gratefully lie down for 10 minutes. One of my clients held me while I sat in the bathroom floor and wretched into the toilet. The amazing thing? She still paid me for that session! It still brings me to tears when I remember all the love they showered upon me.

After 3 chemo treatments, I felt like I was going to die. None of my blood counts were where the doctors wanted them and though they would look at me with empathy and worry, nothing they did was changing anything. I had to make a decision, lose my business or quit chemo. So I did what every logical person would do (add sarcasm here) and I never went back for chemo. Instead, I dedicated 2 hours a day (for the next 7 years mind you, which equals about 5,110 hours) to researching cancer, nutrition, environmental toxins, gut health, stress, sleep, and anything else I could find that may help me achieve true health. I already had a Bachelor's degree in Fitness/Wellness and a Master's degree in Education, but I went back to school to study holistic nutrition, health coaching, neuro-linguistic programming, and hypnosis.

Fast forward to 2018, where I am healthy and have helped many people find their own authentic "healthy." It looks different for each person. That's the beauty of it and also the mystery of it. Health is a process, a journey. It is one of discovering who you really are and then feeding who you were created to be. You have a purpose. You have a mission. And it is unique, so unique that only you can accomplish it. I am thoroughly excited to have you on this journey. I will be praying for you, that you will find your authentic healthy, that you will feel strong and energetic, that you will live out your highest purpose, and that you will in turn bring others to their authentic healthy as well.

Much love and health,

Rhonda

ACKNOWLEDGEMENTS

I must thank the amazing team at Morgan James Publishing. Working with this group of professionals has been one of the best experiences of my life. They have encouraged me, supported me, pushed me, and cared for my own process, my book, and me. Thank you, thank you, thank you!

To my editor, Karen Morgan, you believed in me long before I believed in myself. Thank you for your integrity, attention to detail, and for editing in a way that still allowed me to find and keep my voice and my message. Thank you!

To my daughter, Ashtyn Greene, thank you for designing and running my website all these years. Your assistance with this part of my business has been invaluable. I love you.

To Gary Williams and his team at CX3 Marketing, LLC, thank you for your vision and assistance in pulling together all the many pieces required to consolidate my brand, from the logo to social media to website design. You were professional and a delight to work with!

To Joe Shirey and Mike Hoyt, I can't thank you enough for the countless number of hours you spent helping me streamline my business, set priorities, and maintain my sanity! You both are truly angels on earth!

To Mike Stevans, you provided assistance in any area that was needed, from editing to illustrations to moral support! Thank you! You're amazing!

To Gary Randall of LNR Video Productions, thank you for guiding and directing the production of my online video content! It was a delight working with you!

INTRODUCTION

Welcome to the first step in creating a new and healthier you! Here are two guidelines to help you get the most out of this book.

Before each chapter is a "Chapter Prep." This is an important step, as you will be reviewing things you learned during the prior chapter and you will be setting up habits to help with the next chapter. I encourage you to take your time and get really comfortable with the prep before continuing to the main chapter.

Each chapter has a corresponding video lesson where I will lead you through one of the four sections of that chapter. This is an opportunity for you to connect with me but also for me to add extra guidance on a topic that may be difficult to fully understand from the written version only. These videos will be on my website at www.rhondahuff.com and will be labeled by the Chapter Name, such as "Chapter A."

CHAPTER A PREP

As you begin this important journey to health, here are three important principles that will keep you grounded, focused, and true.

First, Be Authentic with Your Journey

Healing takes place where truth resides. Sometimes it is hard to face and accept the truth but if you want to change and grow, it is essential. Any time you feel like you want to hide or lie to yourself, step into truth instead. It may be hard, you may temporarily feel defeated, you may cry, you may scream, and all of that is ok. Only the truth will get you to your desired goals.

Second, Be Bold Enough To Stop Hiding From Yourself

Your life's purpose requires you, not a poor copy of someone else. Social media is such a great way to stay connected to others but is often a horrible way to stay connected to your own life. It is almost impossible not to get caught up in someone else's "perfect" depiction of their life. If you find that social media is preventing you from staying authentic and bold, consider taking a break from it until you are further along in your journey.

Third, Find Your Center

A mind at peace is stronger than the forces around you. Take time everyday to find your center. This can be done through prayer or meditation. Sometimes even closing your eyes and reciting the word "peace" can help bring calmness to your spirit. This journey may at times take you outside of your comfort zone. When that happens, take a deep breath and reclaim your peace. And once again, remember that this is a process and how long the process takes is totally up to you. Take the time you need and go at a pace that allows you to absorb, practice, and grow.

Before you dig into Chapter A, I want you to simply get curious about your emotions. Record your emotions each day and get curious. What is the emotion cueing you to do? Go ahead and take a stab at it. The muscle used here is discernment, and it takes practice, so be kind to yourself. And remember, honesty outweighs perfection.

My emotions are cues to pay attention.

Emotion	Possible cue

CHAPTER A

Emotional Health

Affirmations

The Latin word for affirm is affirmare, which means "to make firm."

Good health must be built on a firm foundation and that is exactly why we are starting our journey here, by learning to do affirmations.

Let's begin with this one:

I fully love and accept you just as you are right now.

Are you able to say that and mean it? Some people report great difficulty in just saying these words, much less truly meaning them. So how can you get to a point of receiving affirmations that you may not yet believe? By desiring to make them FIRM. When you do, you are saying you choose to love and accept yourself regardless of how your mind/body/heart feels at the moment and regardless of what society/friends/family/enemies may say.

For the next seven days, I want you to tape off a mirror so all that you see are your eyes.

Everyday upon awakening and before retiring, look yourself in the eyes and say seven times, "I fully love and accept you just as you are right now."

Whatever emotions this causes for you is normal. Some people cry, some laugh, and some even get angry. Record here the emotion you feel. Recognize the emotion and get curious about it. Be authentic with yourself. There is a specific reason for your reaction. Let's figure out what it is. I have given an example.

Date	Morning	Emotion	Evening	Emotion	Reasons for these emotions
1/31	7 a.m.	sadness	10 p.m.	anger	Sadness because I don't feel like I mean it. Anger because I don't feel like I deserve it.

Nutritional Health

Add More Green

Throughout the next week eat a handful of green vegetables before anything else goes into your mouth. Yes, that means breakfast too. As long as it is a green vegetable, it counts; so, if celery is the only green vegetable you can stomach right now, eat celery. And that 2 p.m. candy bar craving? Same rule applies. Eat the veggies and then have your candy. How many nutritionists have ever allowed you to keep your candy? Hmmm, there must be a method to her madness…

BLOOD THINNER CAUTION: The best choices are dark green leafy vegetables unless you are on a blood thinner (anticoagulant). If you are on a blood thinner, consult your physician before eating greens that are high in Vitamin K (a natural coagulant). The Mayo Clinic reports that the adequate intake level of vitamin K for people on blood thinners is 120 mcg for adult men and 90 mcg for adult women. While eating small amounts of foods that are rich in vitamin K shouldn't cause a problem, avoid eating large amounts of:

- Kale
- Spinach
- Brussels sprouts
- Parsley
- Collard greens
- Mustard greens
- Chard

Please use this handy chart to record your food.

Time	Green Vegetable	Post-veggie Food(s)

Physical Health

Active Release/Trigger Point Therapy/Self Myofascial Release

Check out www.rhondahuff.com for the video lesson, "Chapter A"

Where there is pain there are nasty little things called *trigger points*. A trigger point is a contracture within an individual muscle fiber. When these contractures refuse to relax, they cause shortening of the muscle which then pulls on connective tissue and joints causing pain. Release the trigger point and you will release much (and many times ALL) of the pain. This is great news as trigger points are very predictable and once you learn how to coerce them to surrender, you have power over pain at your fingertips.

A few nuggets of wisdom:

1. Unless there was an acute injury, the spot where the pain is located is NOT usually where the problem lies. Trigger points refer pain to other places. Sneaky little buggers they are!
2. When you have pain, press areas around and away from the pain point. Usually you will be traveling proximally, which means "closer to the center of the body." So, if the pain is in the wrist, you check the forearms. If the pain is in the front of the knee, you check the quadriceps. The trigger points will feel like small (or sometimes large) painful bumps in the muscle but first they may feel like areas of unusual tightness (until you can loosen them up enough to find the "bumps").
3. Begin by pressing on a sore spot you find. Holding the spot temporarily stops oxygen flow so that when you release it, more healing oxygen flows to the area. It's like giving your muscle an oxygen treatment. Ahhhh!
4. If holding and releasing doesn't work, try different strokes: circular, vertical, horizontal. They can be stubborn so don't let them off the hook too easily. If you begin to feel tingling or numbness, stop and move to a new spot.
5. If you have consistent, chronic pain or sustain an acute injury, consult your physician.

Fascia is connective tissue. It is the biological glue that holds us together. It is essential in understanding the dance between stability and mobility. You can technically think of having one huge muscle that is in 600 fascial pockets. When looking at the body this way, one can see that all movement is synergistic. A problem with the big toe can cause a headache.

By getting proficient at foam rolling and self-myofascial release, you are showing some love to your fascia and your muscles. Poor posture, sitting too long, and injuries are just a few situations that cause the fascia to become more efficient at staying in bad positions. It is the body's attempt to make things easier. For example, someone who works on a computer all day and is sitting in a rounded position requires a lot of energy. Therefore, the body conserves energy by rearranging the fascia to actually help you stay in that rounded position more easily. Then when you try to sit up straight, it is almost impossible to do. Foam rolling followed by proper training can help you regain good posture.

The video will show ways to keep life-giving oxygen flowing properly to the muscles, thus helping to keep trigger points at bay. Do these exercises at least once daily. If you really want to feel change, do them twice daily. Make sure your muscles are warmed up before you foam roll. This can be achieved by simply moving around to get the blood flowing.

Cognitive Health

ABC…ZYX

Recite your ABCs in reverse order from memory! Keep practicing until you can recite them backward as smoothly and effortlessly as forward.

How did you do? Record below.

I mastered my ZYXs in _____ days!!!

CHAPTER B PREP

As you move into Chapter B, it is essential that you continue these habits: speaking affirmations, adding some green, and actively releasing trigger points.

1. Continue Chapter A's affirmation.
   I fully love and accept you just as you are right now.
2. Begin Chapter B's affirmation (still to be done looking only at your eyes, repeating seven times each, morning and night).
   Every part of my body is energized when I breathe.
3. Continue eating a green vegetable before you put anything else in your mouth.
4. Continue foam rolling one or two times a day. This is extremely important for Chapter C's physical health segment.

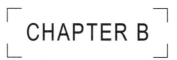

CHAPTER B

Emotional Health

Breathe

Check out www.rhondahuff.com for the video lesson, "Chapter B"

Has anyone ever said to you, "just breathe" when you were going through a tough time or when you were angry about something? Has anyone ever told you that a possible reason of your consistent fatigue is that you aren't breathing properly? What is the big deal with breathing? Isn't that a function of the autonomic nervous system? Doesn't the body breathe just fine without being trained? The answer is a resounding NO!

The effects of proper breathing go far beyond the physical exchange of air in and out of the body. Respiration occurs within the individual cells of the body. Within these cells nutrient fuel is burned with oxygen to release energy to the rest of the body. The nose, trachea, lungs, circulatory system, and muscles play a critical role in determining oxygen supply, and therefore the amount of energy available for everyday life.

About 90 percent of Americans are chest breathers, meaning we only use the top third of our lung capacity. Also, smoking, asthma, and just living in a polluted environment can create scar tissue in the lungs. Once you increase your lung capacity you will also positively affect your energy levels and other bodily functions such as metabolic rate, digestion, and elimination.

For the breathing video, find a room with a comfortable temperature, not too cold or too hot. Blow your nose before you start, sit comfortably, and keep your chin level or slightly down, never allowing it to lift toward the ceiling.

Today's video will teach you a couple of simple techniques that will give you more energy, help you wake up, and help you go to sleep. There are just so many benefits of proper breathing.

Nutritional Health

Build a Better Plan

Nutrition is one of the most confusing aspects of health. Science seems to say one thing today and the opposite thing tomorrow. Think about it this way…who in the world is exactly like you? No one, right? Even identical twins do not have 100 percent of the same genome. Frederick Bieber, a geneticist at Harvard says, "Maybe we shouldn't call them identical twins. We should call them one-egg twins."

Nutrition is as individual as your genome, which is 3.1 billion DNA base pairs. And while it is true that 99.9 percent of humans share the same genome, do you realize how many bits of information that .1 percent happens to be? 3,100,000! How in the world can we expect everyone to react to food in the same way when over 3 million of our DNA base pairs are unique to us? And this doesn't even account for the influence of external environments.

In later chapters we will discuss in detail why certain foods are controversial, but right now I want you to focus on a few basics. I want you to get to know yourself as it relates to nutrition and your mental, emotional, and physical health. I want you to sit with this and be real with this and apply this. Revelations may come in days, weeks, or months. Do this for yourself and take the time you need. This is an oxygen mask and you must save yourself first. Don't point fingers or think about who else needs this right now. YOU need this right now. Saving others can come later.

In a journal or on a piece of paper, write these headings and do this exercise for at least seven days. Please commit to continuing the exercise until you begin to see a correlation develop. When I do this exercise with people face-to-face, I highlight any common foods that were eaten on days where similar symptoms were present. For example, if red meat or tomatoes were often present on the same days that the client reported aching joints then I highlighted those foods. If you like to figure out things you will enjoy this activity. But even if you don't, it is important to your success moving forward so dig in your heels and make it happen for your own sake.

Today's Date:

Pain I have TODAY:

_____

_____

_____

_____

Emotions I have TODAY:

_____

_____

_____

_____

Cognitive issues (such as brain fog, not finding words, etc.) I have TODAY:

_____

_____

_____

_____

Food I ate YESTERDAY:

_____

_____

_____

_____

At the very end when you begin to see these correlations, record it like this: Potential problematic foods for my individual makeup are:

_____

_____

_____

_____

I bet you can guess why I chose that wording. If you guessed, "she is reiterating that no one else is like me, and my nutritional needs may be completely different from everyone else's" then you are exactly right!

Now the ball is in your court. Be bold enough and brave enough to begin eliminating these foods from your nutritional plan. Will it be easy? Probably not. Will it be worth it? You bet your sweet caramel-coated popcorn it will!

Physical Health

Bedtime

Some of the biggest complaints I hear from people involves the lack of proper sleep: can't go to sleep, can't stay asleep, can't wake up, can't stay awake, a spouse's snoring/talking/thrashing about prevents sleep, and the list goes on. Chances are, you are nodding your head right now.

Recently, sleep has been touted as one health practice that you simply can't afford to ignore. It is important for absolutely any health goal you have, whether it's to lose weight, have more energy, decrease stress, reduce blood pressure, protect your heart, refresh your mind, improve your memory, decrease depression, decrease anxiety, curb inflammation, decrease pain, improve focus, or even to live longer. That's right! All of these can be directly related to sleep. And the key is in the *quality*.

So, what is happening while we sleep anyway? Here is a synopsis.

Sleep is part of what is considered the "circadian (which means 'about a day') rhythm" of life. Your brain wants to sleep when it gets dark and awaken when it gets light. This was very effective before the invention of electricity. People would go to sleep and wake up with the rhythm of nature. They'd sleep when it was dark, work when it was light. But now we stay awake long after dark and often must wake up before daylight. It totally throws our natural circadian rhythm out of balance. According to Ayurvedic medicine, the most restorative sleep happens between 10 p.m. and 2 a.m. Try to sleep most nights during those hours.

The Five Stages of Sleep:
Stage 1—Light Sleep
- Lasts about seven minutes
- Alpha and theta brain waves
- Begin to drift in and out of sleep
- Muscles relax and muscle activity slows

- Eyes move slowly
- Easily awakened
- Typical ratio of overall sleep: 5 percent to 15 percent

Stage 2—Light Sleep

- Lasts about twenty minutes
- Brain waves become slower with only occasional bursts of rapid brain waves called sleep spindles
- Eye movements stop
- Breathing and heart rate slow down
- Typical ratio of overall sleep: 50 percent

Stage 3 and Stage 4—Deep (Delta) Sleep

- In Stage 3 extremely slow brain waves (delta waves) are interspersed with smaller, faster waves and is a transitional period between Stage 2 and Stage 4.
- In Stage 4, the brain produces primarily delta waves. It lasts about thirty minutes.
- Heart rate and breathing slow further
- No body or eye movements
- The brain is resting now. You don't dream.
- It is very difficult to wake a person in sleep Stage 3 and Stage 4.
- This is repair time for the body. Your kidneys clean your blood, your hormones reset, your organs detox, your cells are replaced, your wounds heal, and your muscle tissue rebuilds.
- If awakened during either stage, you will feel very groggy or disoriented.
- Bedwetting, night terrors, and sleepwalking happen during Stage 3 and Stage 4.
- Typical ratio of overall sleep: 5 percent to 15 percent

Stage 5—REM (Rapid Eye Movement) Sleep

- Brain becomes active again. It's as active as when you are awake, and you dream intensively during this stage.
- Hormones are released that put you in a narcotic state so the limbs are temporarily paralyzed (otherwise you would act out your dreams).
- The first REM cycle of the night lasts about ten minutes but gets longer each cycle and may last up to an hour by the last REM cycle of the night.
- Breathing becomes rapid, irregular, and shallow
- Brain and body are energized
- Heart rate increases

- Blood pressure rises
- Helps store memories and balance moods
- If you are awakened during REM sleep, you can remember your dream.
- Most people experience three to five intervals of REM sleep per night.
- Typical ratio of overall sleep: 20 percent to 25 percent for adults (50 percent for infants!)

Sleep's Role

- Improves and strengthens memory through a process called "consolidation," which allows you to "practice" what you are learning.
- Curbs inflammation. People who get less than six hours of sleep have higher levels of inflammatory proteins, such as C-reactive protein which increases heart attack risk
- Promotes a healthy body composition. During weight loss, those who are sleep-deprived lose more muscle and those with adequate sleep lose more fat.
- Keeps hormones in balance. Sleep and metabolism are controlled by the same sectors of the brain. When you are sleepy certain hormones go up in your blood. Those same hormones drive appetite.
- Helps us deal with stress more effectively.
- Staves off depression/anxiety. Those who are sleep-deprived tend to struggle more with depression and anxiety.
- Sleep cannot be "made up" on the weekends.

Tips for Better Sleep

- Cut out late-night caffeine
- Cut out late-night alcohol (alcohol can help you fall asleep but is proven to cause restless and incomplete sleep patterns, never allowing your body to fully recover)
- Keep the room dark. Melatonin is produced in the pineal gland. This happens naturally once the sun goes down and stays in the blood stream for about twelve hours. When we keep lights on (including TVs, computers, and bright reading lights) it inhibits the release of melatonin. This makes it hard to fall asleep and hard to wake up since it stays in our bloodstream for about twelve hours. And, unfortunately, it has not been proven that melatonin supplements are safe long term

- Keep the temperature slightly cool
- Keep electronics out of the bedroom (even the smallest light from your computer can trigger your brain to wake up)
- Keep work out of the bedroom (the bedroom should be used for sleep and sex)
- Have a bedtime ritual. Remember childhood?
- Practice the breath work from this chapter's *Emotional Health* segment
- Check to see which nostril is open and which is closed. The right nostril is "awake" and the left nostril is "asleep." If the left nostril is stopped up, plug the right nostril and force the left one to open. It will induce sleep.
- Listen to Delta Sleep Music (free music on YouTube. I like the eight-hour ones)
- Have a pen and paper on your nightstand to write down things that are on your mind. It allows the mind to trust that it won't be forgotten
- Write early morning pages. As soon as you wake up, write down everything you can remember about your dreams and thoughts. Dreams help us find solutions. Watch for patterns and ideas to emerge.

I would like for you to track your sleep for the next seven days. If you have a fitness tracker with a sleep-tracking feature, you can use that. Otherwise download a free app on your phone and then you will lay the phone on the bed next to you. Unfortunately, you need to sleep alone with this option because it will pick up your partner's movements as well. The way it works is by monitoring when you are moving and when you are not. Please know that this is going to be a raw estimation. No device is going to work perfectly.

As you read above, the Deep (Delta and REM) Sleep is when you are not moving and that should be about 5 percent to 15 percent and 20 percent to 25 percent respectively (25 percent to 40 percent combined) of your night's sleep. Therefore, if you get the recommended amount of sleep of seven to nine hours (for adults), that means your deep sleep should look similar to this chart:

Hours Slept	Deep Sleep	Other Sleep
7	1.75–2.8 hours	4.2–5.25 hours
8	2–3.2 hours	4.8–5.7 hours
9	2.25–3.6 hours	5.4–6.75 hours

This is your chart. Please fill in for seven days.

Day	Hours Slept	Deep Sleep	Other Sleep	Sleep Tips Used
1				
2				
3				
4				
5				
6				
7				

This is what I learned about my sleep patterns in this exercise.

_____

_____

_____

_____

This is what I will do to ensure proper sleep going forward.

_____

_____

_____

_____

Cognitive Health

Brain Food

Omega-3 fats can help lower your risk of heart disease, cognitive decline, auto-immune disease, Crohn's disease, Parkinson's disease, osteoporosis, rheumatoid arthritis, breast cancer, prostate cancer, depression, hypertension, diabetes, obesity, premature aging, and ADHD.

Omega-3s are called *essential* fatty acids because the body cannot make them.

There are different types of omega-3s:

- DHA (docosahexaenoic acid)
- EPA (eicosapentaenoic acid)

- ALA (alpha-linolenic acid)—Your body can turn the ALA from plant sources into EPA, though not very efficiently. Only 5 percent to 10 percent will convert to EPA if your gut is already in good health.

Americans typically eat too many omega-6 fats in food products sourced from corn, soy, canola, safflower, and sunflower oils. The ideal ratio of omega-6 to omega-3 fats is 1:1 to 4:1. The Standard American Diet (SAD) averages from 20:1 to 50:1. This is a serious problem because omega-6 fats encourage the production of inflammation in the body.

Research from the Institute for Functional Medicine shows that therapeutic doses of EPA/DHA work as well as Cox 1 (aspirin, ibuprophen, naproxen) and Cox 2 (Celebrex, Vioxxc, Bextra) inhibitors and without the negative side effects.

The EPA to DHA ratio should be 1.5:1.

For inflammatory diseases, such as Alzheimer's, arthritis, diabetes, depression, GERD, infections, multiple chemical sensitivity, psoriasis, eczema, colitis, arthritis, cancer, atherosclerosis, etc. and auto-immune diseases, such as lupus, Sjogren's, dermatitis, fibromyalgia, celiac, Crohn's, Hashimoto's thyroiditis, IBD/IBS, lyme disease, myasthenia gravis, multiple sclerosis, peripheral neuropathy, psoriasis, Raynaud's phenomenon, sarcoidosis, scleroderma, type 1 diabetes, ulcerative colitis, vitiligo, etc., the dosage recommendations are 3 grams to 6 grams total combined per day. Remember the 1.5:1 ration of EPA:DHA. (Less than 1.5 grams and more than 7 grams have proven to be ineffective). It is important to build up to these amounts gradually.

IMPORTANT: If your doctor already has you on an omega-3 supplement, please continue its use. If you are on anticoagulants, please consult your doctor before increasing your intake of omega-3 fats.

Food Sources of Omega-3 Fats

Fish: Although you could get all the omega-3s you would ever need from fish, there is a problem. The majority of the fish supply is heavily tainted with industrial toxins, such as heavy metals, PCBs, and radioactive poisons. And the highest concentrations of mercury are found in the large, carnivorous fish like tuna, sea bass, swordfish, and marlin. Also, be sure to avoid farmed salmon, which contains half the omega-3 as wild and hosts a range of contaminants such as harmful metabolic byproducts and agricultural residues from the GMO corn- and soy-based feed they are given. The weekly recommendation for a healthy adult (who is NOT pregnant) is seven ounces. This by itself won't provide enough omega-3 fats.

Safe fish: wild-caught Alaskan salmon and very small fish like sardines.

Fish oil: Fish oil is among the primary ways that people supplement their intake of omega-3 fats. Even high-quality fish oils are weak in antioxidants. So, you actually increase the need for added antioxidant protection. This happens because fish oil is a bit perishable, and oxidation leads to the formation of harmful free radicals. Antioxidants are, therefore, necessary to ensure that the fish oil doesn't oxidize and become rancid in your body. If you are burping fish, it is already rancid and you should throw it out.

Cod liver oil: Research from the University of California, Berkley, warns that cod liver oil may cause birth defects and weaken bones due to the high amount of vitamin A it contains.

Krill oil: The antioxidant potency is forty-eight times higher than fish oil. It also contains natural astaxanthin, a marine-source flavonoid that creates a special bond with the EPA and DHA to allow direct metabolism of the antioxidants, making them more bioavailable. Therefore, you get more assimilation, even though it contains less EPA and DHA than other fish. Another great thing is that there has never been a krill shortage forecasted.

Meat and dairy from grass-fed animals, and enriched or pastured eggs also contain some EPA/DHA

Kale, spinach, walnuts, chia seeds, flax seeds, and hemp seeds contain ALA, some of which the body converts to EPA, but only about 5 percent to 10 percent.

If you are on an anticoagulant, please discuss omega-3 supplementation with your physician.

The American Heart Association recommends 1000 mg per day of DHA/EPA to lower the risk of heart disease and 2000 to 4000 mg per day of DHA/EPA to lower triglycerides. Consult your physician for exact dosages.

Food	Serving size	Amount of Omega-3s per serving	Weekly intake
Mackerel, DHA/EPA	3.5 oz (palm size)	5134 mg	
Wild-caught Alaskan salmon, DHA/EPA	3.5 oz (palm size)	2260 mg	
Herring, DHA/EPA	3.5 oz (palm size)	1729 mg	
Sardines, DHA/EPA	3.5 oz	1480 mg	
Anchovies, DHA/EPA	2 oz.	951 mg	
Oysters, DHA/EPA	6 oysters	565 mg	
Chia seeds—ALA—converts to EPA more efficiently than flax seeds	1 oz	4915 mg	
Walnuts, ALA	7 walnuts	2542 mg	
Flax seeds (ground), ALA	1 tbsp ground	2338 mg	
Spinach, ALA	1 cup cooked	352 mg	
Raw wild rice, ALA	½ cup	240 mg	
Cauliflower, ALA	1 cup cooked	208 mg	
Brussels sprouts, ALA	½ cup cooked	135 mg	
Kale, ALA	1 cup raw	121 mg	
Pastured/enriched eggs, ALA	1 egg	115 mg	
Grass-fed dairy, ALA	8 oz	100 mg	
Grass-fed meat, ALA	3.5 oz	80 mg	

The above listed foods have good ratios of Omega 6 to Omega 3 fats. Remember that Omega 6 fats are inflammatory, and some nuts and all grain-fed beef and dairy products are very high in them.

Here are a few more EPA/DHA safety and sustainability resources.

Metallo and organotoxins in fish:

www.edf.org

www.epa.gov

www.ewg.org

www.fishoilsafety.com

Sustainability:

www.mbari.org

www.marinebio.org

www.lighthouse-foundation.org

www.wholefoodsmarket.com

CHAPTER C PREP

1. Continue Chapter A's affirmation until you believe it.
   I fully love and accept you just as you are right now.
2. Begin Chapter C's affirmation (still to be done looking only at your eyes, repeating seven times each, morning and night).
   I am open to positive change in all areas of my life.
3. Continue eating a green vegetable before you put anything else in your mouth. Begin working toward spacing meals four to five hours apart. Do not stress out about this. Start slowly and keep moving forward as we begin regulating insulin/leptin levels.
4. Foam roll before doing the corrective exercises in this chapter's *Physical Health* segment.
5. Continue practicing deep breathing.
6. Continue to monitor your sleep quality and experiment with the tools given in the last chapter until you find something that works. Record the things that are working for you:

   _____
   _____
   _____

CHAPTER C

Emotional Health

Circle of Life

The Circle of Life exercise is used to assess PRIMARY FOOD© and was developed by Joshua Rosenthal at the Institute for Integrative Nutrition. Primary foods are relationships, career, spirituality, and physical activity. When any of these areas are out of balance, you will turn to secondary foods (the actual food you put into your mouth). Look at each section of the circle and place a dot on the line marking how satisfied you are with each area of your life. A dot placed closer to the inside indicates dissatisfaction, while a dot placed on the periphery indicates ultimate happiness. Dots placed right in the middle may indicate that you do not know yourself well enough or you are dealing with some form of denial so try to decide if you are more satisfied or less satisfied than a middle of the road score. When you have placed a dot on each of the lines, connect the dots to see your circle of life. You will have a clear visual of any imbalances in primary food and a starting point for determining where you may wish to spend more time and energy to create balance and joy in your life.

Once you have connected the dots, take a close look at the three lowest scores and answer the questions below:

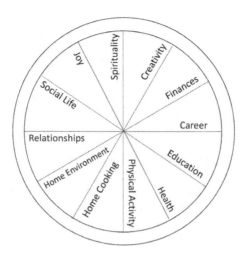

What is ranked Number 12?

_____

_____

Why am I unhappy with this area of my life?

_____

_____

Here is one action step I will take this week to enhance my happiness in this area:

_____

_____

What is ranked Number 11?

_____

_____

Why am I unhappy with this area of my life?

_____

_____

Here is one action step I will take this week to enhance my happiness in this area:

_____

_____

What is ranked Number 10?

_____

_____

Why am I unhappy with this area of my life?

_____

_____

Here is one action step I will take this week to enhance my happiness in this area:

_____

_____

Nutritional Health

Cravings
Primary Causes of Cravings

1. **Lack of primary food.** Being dissatisfied with a relationship or having an inappropriate exercise routine (too much, too little or the wrong type), being bored, stressed, uninspired by a job, or lacking a spiritual practice may all cause emotional eating. Eating can be used as a substitute for entertainment or to fill the void of insufficient primary food. The Circle of Life exercise in this chapter's Emotional Health section is designed to help you uncover areas of potential to help you increase satisfaction levels in all areas of your life.

2. **Lack of water.** Lack of water can send the message that you are thirsty and on the verge of dehydration. Dehydration can manifest as a mild hunger, so the first thing to do when you get a craving is drink a full glass of water. What people don't realize, however, is that excess water can also cause cravings, so be sure that your water intake is well balanced. A good rule of thumb is to take your weight and divide by two to determine how many ounces of water you need per day. You then adjust the amount as needed. For example, if you are in the sun or having a heavy workout day you may need more and on less active days you may need less. The key is to listen to your body.

3. **Yin/yang imbalance.** Certain foods have more yin qualities (expansive) while other foods have more yang qualities (contractive). Eating foods that are either extremely yin or extremely yang causes cravings in order to maintain balance.

For example, eating a diet too rich in sugar (yin) may cause a craving for meat (yang). Eating too many raw foods (yin) may cause cravings for extremely cooked (dehydrated) foods or vice versa.

4. **Inside coming out.** Often cravings come from foods that we have recently eaten, foods eaten by our ancestors, or foods from our childhood. It is not uncommon for people to get strange cravings of foods they have never eaten, only to realize it is a food of their ancestors. A clever way to satisfy these cravings is to eat a healthier version of one's ancestral or childhood foods.

5. **Seasons.** Often the body craves foods that balance the elements of the season. In the spring, people crave detoxifying foods like leafy greens or citrus foods. In the summer, people crave cooling foods like fruit, raw foods and ice cream, and in the fall, people crave grounding foods like squash, onions and nuts. During winter, many crave hot and heat-producing foods like meat, oil and fat. Holidays can trigger cravings for particular foods like turkey, eggnog or sweets.

6. **Lack of nutrients.** If the body has inadequate nutrients, it will produce odd cravings. For example, inadequate mineral levels produce salt cravings, and overall inadequate nutrition produces cravings for non-nutritional forms of energy, like caffeine.

7. **Hormones.** When women experience menstruation, pregnancy or menopause, fluctuating testosterone and estrogen levels may cause unique cravings.

8. **De-evolution.** When things are going extremely well, sometimes a self-sabotage syndrome happens. We crave foods that throw us off, thus creating more cravings to balance ourselves. This often happens from low blood sugar and may result in strong mood swings. To recognize an episode of self-sabotage is extremely important. Always remember that the point is progress not perfection. Sometimes we can be just as afraid of success as we are of failure. Recognize it, plan for it, and conquer it.

What Are Your Cravings Telling You?

Sugar
- "I need energy! And fast!"
  - ✓ Eat kale, raw cacao beans/nibs, broccoli, hemp seeds, berries

Salt
- "I need minerals!"
  - ✓ Eat seaweed, such as spirulina, wakame, nori, kombu, arame

Crunchy
- "I am so frustrated/angry right now!"
  - ✓ Eat carrots, bell peppers, apples, nuts, seeds

Creamy
- "I feel so unappreciated."
  - ✓ Probably you just need a hug! But try avocado, Greek yogurt, or a baked sweet potato

I can relate to these cravings:	I will try this:	Did it work?

Physical Health

Corrective Exercise

Check out www.rhondahuff.com for the video lesson, "Chapter C"

Corrective exercise is a crucial part of safely and effectively getting into shape.

According to renowned physical therapist, Gray Cook, "The rule is this: Mobility before stability, stability before movement, and movement before strength."

This segment is designed to restore proper mobility/stability in your body. The last two chapters have focused on self-myofascial release, which has prepared your body for the upcoming corrective work.

The body alternates joint mobility with joint stability. This means that the feet should be stable, the ankles should be mobile, the knees should be stable, the hips mobile, the lumbar spine stable, the t-spine mobile, the scapula stable, the shoulder joint mobile, the lower cervical spine stable, and the upper cervical spine mobile. Our correctives are specifically designed to facilitate achieving the proper mobility and stability for your joints. Do ten repetitions for each corrective.

In this video you will learn some of the basic corrective exercises to improve total body movement, which is one of the most important aspects of staying functional and healthy. The chart below gives you the three different correctives workouts. You are free to pick your own skip day. I just put the day off in the middle on day four.

Remember to foam roll BEFORE doing the correctives.

CORRECTIVES	Days 1 and 5	10 Reps per Side	
Foot Stability	Towel drags or marble pick-ups		
Ankle Mobility	Wall ankle mobility		
Knee Stability	Knee extension to leg raise	Seated	Standing
Hip Mobility	Supine alternating Spiderman stretch		
Lumbar Stability	Abdominal corrections		
Thoracic Spine Mobility	Side-lying rotations with reach		
Scapular Stability	No money exercise		
Shoulder Mobility	Floor angel or wall angel		
Lower Cervical Stability	Head-backs		
Upper Cervical Mobility	Cervical side bending		

CORRECTIVES	DAYS 2 and 6	10 Reps per Side	
Foot Stability	One leg stand		
Ankle Mobility	Toes up/heels up		
Knee Stability	Sit to stand squats		
Hip Mobility	Piriformis pulse and stretch	Seated	Supine
Lumbar Stability	Active leg lowering	Leg bent	Leg straight
Thoracic Spine Mobility	Thoracic opener with dowel		
Scapular Stability	Wall slides to high V with lift off		
Shoulder Mobility	Shoulder dislocates with dowel		

Lower Cervical Stability	Hand to head press	Front	Sides	Back
Upper Cervical Mobility	Cervical rotations			

CORRECTIVES	DAYS 3 and 7	10 Reps per Side
Foot Stability	Transverse step to balance	
Ankle Mobility	Flexed-knee 3-way ankle mobility matrix	
Knee Stability	Step ups with glute focus	
Hip Mobility	Seated internal and external hip rotations (windshield wipers)	
Lumbar Stability	Quadruped chops	
Thoracic Spine Mobility	Quadruped T-spine rotation with lumbar lock	
Scapular Stability	Band pull-aparts	
Shoulder Mobility	Wall sit dorsiflexion with unilateral reach—dowel	
Lower Cervical Stability	Prone and supine head holds	
Upper Cervical Mobility	Diagonal exercises	

Cognitive Health

Crosswords

For the next seven days, set a timer for ten minutes and see how much of a crossword puzzle you can complete. The goal is **speed**.

How did you do?

_____

_____

_____

Did your speed improve each day?

CHAPTER D PREP

1. Continue Chapter A's affirmation until you believe it.
   I fully love and accept you just as you are right now.
2. Begin Chapter D's affirmation (still to be done looking only at your eyes, repeating seven times each, morning and night).
   I choose to stay calm in moments of stress.
3. If cravings are still a struggle, continue to experiment with the cravings segment from Chapter C.
4. Foam roll before doing the corrective exercises from Chapter C's *Physical Health* segment.
5. Continue practicing deep breathing.
6. If sleep is still an issue, continue to monitor your sleep quality and experiment with the tools provided until you find something that works. If you have found something, record it here.

   _____
   _____
   _____

7. Work your Circle of Life action steps and record your progress below:

   _____
   _____
   _____

CHAPTER D

Emotional Health

Distress or Eustress?

The pioneering Hungarian-Canadian endocrinologist Hans Selye coined the term "stress" in 1936 and defined it as "the nonspecific response of the body to any demand for change." Stress very quickly became a buzzword, but unfortunately Selye's true meaning was ignored. As a matter of fact, the Oxford English Dictionary defines stress as "a state of mental or emotional strain or tension resulting from adverse or demanding circumstances." This was not Selye's definition.

Selye made a clear distinction between what he called eustress (good stress) and distress (bad stress) and used the "Human Function Curve" to demonstrate the difference. (See next page for diagram)

What is Stress?

- **Distress**: physical, mental, or emotional **tension** that leads to a perception that the demands exceed the personal and social resources the individual is able to mobilize. This causes lost productivity and illness. Kansas State University psychology professor and author Dr. David Danskin estimates that 85 percent of doctor visits are due to stress-related causes.

Stress Curve

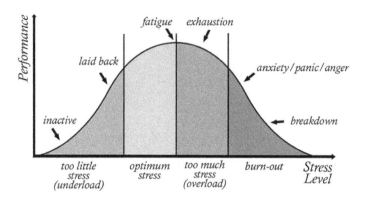

- **Eustress**: physical, mental, or emotional **motivation** that leads to increased productivity and well-being.

We need a healthy level of stress in order to get out of bed and be productive human beings. It is only when you cross from healthy stress (eustress) to unhealthy stress (distress) that your health and performance becomes negatively affected.

How to Know When You Have Gone Over the Edge
- Anger, temper flares, mood swings
- Depression
- Food or drink issues
- Weight changes
- Forgetfulness
- Obsessiveness
- Shunning social activities or sex
- Sleep disturbances, fatigue, no energy

Once you have gone over the hump of maximum activity and reached the stress zone, all sorts of issues can surface. A very common issue is adrenal fatigue. The adrenals are small glands located on top of the kidneys. The adrenal glands produce hormones that help control heart rate, blood pressure, how well the body turns food into energy, the levels of minerals in the blood, and other functions particularly involved in stress reactions. Those stress reactions are our focus. Take a moment to circle any symptoms you are currently having.

The hypothalamus, pituitary, adrenal (HPA) axis is the body's central stress response system. The Institute of Functional Medicine uses this questionnaire with permission from wholepsychiatry.com to help assess and differentiate dysfunction within this system. The goal of the exercise is to obtain and collate data that will give you an idea of the presence and type of a possible HPA axis dysfunction. These symptoms and signs are primarily a compilation from the *Williams Textbook of Endocrinology—11th edition*, as well as recent literature, and lastly, clinical experience.

Please score only the items you are currently experiencing on a scale of one to four:

1. This is a mild problem
2. This is a significant problem
3. This is a major problem
4. This is a severe problem

Low Cortisol State

1. ____Lethargic depression
2. ____Excessive need for sleep
3. ____Chronic fatigue syndrome
4. ____Chronic pain
5. ____Fibromyalgia (musculoskeletal tender points)
6. ____Dizziness when you stand or bend
7. ____Low blood pressure and/or drop of blood pressure on standing
8. ____Craving salty foods-pretzels, pickles etc.
9. ____Poor wound healing
10. ____Easy bruising
11. ____Fatigue
12. ____Inability to handle even slight stresses
13. ____Hypoglycemia: dizzy, irritable, or sleepy if you go without food for four to five hours; symptoms relieved by food
14. ____Scars, elbows, nipples, or skin near nails that are unusually dark
15. ____Slow healing of cuts
16. ____Unstable body temperatures (hot or cold)

Elevated Cortisol State

1. ____Agitated depression
2. ____Weight gain around your abdomen, back of neck, and in the face and cheeks

3. ____Stretch marks not from weight loss
4. ____Adult onset diabetes
5. ____Osteoporosis
6. ____Craving sweets
7. ____Trouble falling or staying asleep

Adrenal Hyperplasia
1. ____Excessive dark male pattern hair growth (women)
2. ____Irregular or no periods (not menopausal)
3. ____Eastern European heritage

Add up your totals for each section. Enter them below and divide by the indicated highest score for each section. The totals will indicate which areas need focus. Rather than an absolute cutoff to use, there is a continuum between normal and dysfunction. If you are seeing a functional medical provider (to find one in your area go to www.ifm.org/find-a-practitioner/), this information should be used in conjunction with blood testing and salivary cortisol testing.

- Low cortisol state ____/64 = ____
- Elevated cortisol state ____/28 = ____
- Adrenal hyperplasia ____/12 = ___

Nutritional Health

Disordered Eating
Disordered eating, though similar to eating disorders, is different in its scope and severity. If you think you have an actual *eating disorder,* please seek the counsel of a therapist who has experience in this area. I struggled with bulimia from the age of sixteen to age twenty-three and anorexia nervosa from the age of twenty-three to age twenty-six.

I understand how difficult it is to heal from those disorders. Only through professional counseling was I able to deal with the real issues behind the disorders and get well.

Many of the people with whom I have worked had full-blown eating disorders, are currently dealing with an eating disorder, or are struggling with disordered eating. If you have had an eating disorder in your past but are "recovered" you may still struggle with disordered eating. I do. My natural tendency is to skip meals. I actually have a couple of really close friends who hold me accountable to a normal eating pattern. If this is something with which you struggle, I highly recommend having an accountability partner.

What is true hunger? When the stomach rumbles and growls most people assume they are hungry. This is actually not true at all. First of all, the area where people are hearing and feeling this is usually the intestines, not the stomach. What really is happening is your body is trying to digest previously eaten food and/or detoxify the body from processed and pro-inflammatory foods. True hunger happens just below and to the left of the xiphoid process of the sternum in the actual stomach. True hunger will then radiate up the esophagus and be felt in the back of the throat.

Here is a comparison chart of behaviors and attitudes of disordered eating patterns versus healthy eating patterns.

Disordered eating behaviors and attitudes
Binge eating
Dieting
Skipping meals regularly
Self-induced vomiting
Obsessive calorie counting
Self-worth based on body shape and weight
Misusing laxatives or diuretics
Chronic restrained eating
Healthy eating behaviors and attitudes
Eat more on some days, less on others
Eat some foods just because they taste good
Have a positive attitude towards food
Not label foods with judgment words such as "good," "bad," "clean"
Overeat occasionally
Under-eat occasionally
Crave certain foods at times
Treat food and eating as one small part of a balanced life

One area of eating that I do want to address is the "eat several meals throughout the day" mind set. That philosophy was developed for athletes who are working out six to eight hours a day. So, if that fits you, go ahead and eat a ton of meals. If that isn't you, I would like for you to try a different way of eating. We need three solid meals and no snacks.

Oh boy! I hit a nerve, didn't I? Before you toss me in the trash, hear me out. Here is what we know, scientifically.

1. When you eat, insulin is released into the blood stream and stays there for about three and a half hours. Your body can't burn fat in the presence of insulin. Therefore, if you are eating every three hours, you are going to store a lot of fat.

2. Eating too often can cause leptin resistance. Leptin is the gatekeeper of fat metabolism and energy balance in the body. It also regulates hunger and is directly tied to insulin levels. Elevated leptin levels can contribute to high blood pressure, obesity, infertility, premature aging, heart disease, stroke, and diabetes. Healthy leptin levels are best maintained if there is at least a four-hour rest between meals.

3. "Breakfast is the most important meal of the day" was developed by food companies to sell products.

4. According to Ayurveda (the most ancient medical practice in the world) the largest meal should be lunch and consumed between noon and 2 p.m. because that is when our digestive fire is the strongest. So, if you like carbs, eat them at lunch.

5. Ayurveda also suggests that dinner be lighter and consumed before 8 p.m. so it doesn't mess up your sleep. After 10 p.m. the body is working to burn off toxins and continue to digest food from the day. Eating after 10 p.m. will cause toxins to build up and leave you feeling tired in the morning.

6. It is proven that a twelve-hour fast through the night will:
   a. Reduce: blood lipids (including decreased triglycerides and LDL cholesterol), blood pressure, markers of inflammation (including CRP<, IL-6, TNF, BDNF, and more), and oxidative stress (using markers of protein, lipid, and DNA damage)
   b. Increase: cellular turnover and repair (autophagocytosis), fat burning, growth hormone release, and metabolic rate

c. Improve: appetite control (through changes in PPY and ghrelin), blood sugar control (by lowering blood glucose and increasing insulin sensitivity), cardiovascular function (by offering protection against ischemic injury to the heart), and neurogenesis and neuronal plasticity (by offering protection against neurotoxins)

So, let's try to get some of this under control.

IMPORTANT NOTE: If you have diabetes, you will need to lengthen the times between meals SLOWLY and I encourage you to discuss the plan with a functional medicine physician. And do not do an overnight twelve-hour fast without your doctor's permission.

If you do NOT have diabetes, here is your GOAL:

- Finish your last meal by 8 p.m.
- Wait twelve hours before eating breakfast (so if you want to eat breakfast at 7 a.m., finish your last meal the night before by 7 p.m.).
- Wait four hours before eating lunch. Try to eat between noon and 2 p.m. and make it your biggest meal.
- Wait four hours before eating an early dinner or healthy snack

If you are accustomed to grazing, this allows you to eat four times in the course of a day, even though our goal will eventually be only three. If you are already only eating three meals a day, continue to do so but add the above principles to it.

If you are diabetic or pre-diabetic, here is your GOAL but I still recommend that you discuss any and all changes to your lifestyle habits with your physician.

Extend meal times by fifteen to thirty minutes each day (you should not feel light-headed or dizzy). You are working up to at least four hours between meals in the future. Monitor your blood sugar levels and remember to not attempt overnight fasting without your doctor's permission.

The American Diabetic Association states these guidelines on their website:

For people using insulin, the ADA recommends testing three or more times a day. If you take another kind of medication, test your blood sugar level as often as your healthcare team recommends.

Your doctor will determine when you should test your blood sugar based on your current health, age and level of activity, as well as the time of day and other factors. They may suggest that you test your blood sugar at any of the following times:

- Before each meal
- One or two hours after a meal
- Before a bedtime snack
- In the middle of the night
- Before physical activity, to see if you need a snack
- During and after physical activity
- If you think your blood sugar might be too high or too low, or falling
- When you're sick or under stress

Physical Health

Dosha and Exercise

Check out www.rhondahuff.com for the video lesson, "Chapter D"

Just as there is no "one-size-fits-all" for nutrition, the same holds true for exercise. Have you ever wondered why your best friend lost a lot of weight when she started running and when you decided to do the same thing, you felt horrible and started to gain weight? It may be that you are a different dosha type than your friend.

For the five profile tables on the next few pages:

1. Circle the phrase that best describes your qualities for each of the categories in the left-hand column.
2. Tally the number of circles for each column on the subtotal lines at the bottom of each table.
3. Transfer the subtotals for each profile onto the *Grand Totals Table* on the last page.
4. Add up the Grand Totals.

MENTAL PROFILE			
	WINTER/VATA	SUMMER/PITTA	SPRING/KAPHA
Mental activity	Quick mind, restless	Sharp intellect, aggressive	Calm, steady, stable
Memory	Short-term best	Good general memory	Long-term best

Thoughts	Constantly changing	Fairly steady	Steady, stable, fixed
Concentration	Short-term focus best	Better than average mental concentration	Good ability for long-term focus
Ability to learn	Quick grasp of learning	Medium to moderate grasp	Slow to learn new things
Dreams	Fearful, flying, running, jumping	Angry, fiery, violent, adventurous	Include water, clouds, relationships, romance
Sleep	Interrupted, light	Sound, medium	Sound, heavy, long
Speech	Fast, sometimes missing words	Fast, sharp, clear-cut	Slow, clear, sweet
Voice	High pitched	Medium pitched	Low pitched
Mental Subtotal	_____	_____	_____

BEHAVIORAL PROFILE

	WINTER/VATA	SUMMER/PITTA	SPRING/KAPHA
Eating speed	Quick	Medium	Slow
Hunger level	Irregular	Sharp, needs food when hungry	Can easily miss meals
Food and drink	Prefers warm	Prefers cold	Prefers dry and warm
Achieving goals	Easily distracted	Focused and driven	Slow and steady
Giving/donations	Gives small amounts	Gives nothing, or large amounts infrequently	Gives regularly and generously
Relationships	Many casual	Intense	Long and deep
Sex drive	Variable or low	Moderate	Strong
Works best	While supervised	Alone	In groups
Weather preference	Aversion to cold	Aversion to heat	Aversion to damp, cool

Reaction to stress	Excites quickly	Medium	Slow to get excited
Financial	Doesn't save, spends quickly	Saves, but big spender	Saves regularly, accumulates wealth
Friendships	Tends toward short-term friendships, makes friends quickly	Tends to be a loner, friends related to occupation	Tends to form long-lasting friendships
Behavioral Subtotal	_____	_____	_____

PHYSICAL PROFILE

	WINTER/VATA	SUMMER/PITTA	SPRING/KAPHA
Amount of hair	Average	Thinning	Thick
Hair type	Dry	Normal	Oily
Hair color	Light brown, blonde	Red, auburn	Dark brown, black
Skin	Dry, rough, or both	Soft, normal to oily	Oily, moist, cool
Skin temperature	Cold hands/feet	Warm	Cool
Complexion	Darker	Pink-red	Pale-white
Eyes	Small	Medium	Large
Whites of eyes	Blue/brown	Yellow or red	Glossy white
Size of teeth	Very large or very small	Small-medium	Medium-large
Weight	Thin, hard to gain	Medium	Heavy, gains easily
Elimination	Dry, hard, thin, easily constipated	Many during day, soft to normal	Heavy, slow, thick, regular
Resting pulse	Take a full 60-second pulse after waking up naturally (without an alarm clock). Record pulse here:		
Men	70-90	60-70	50-60
Women	80-100	70-80	60-70

Veins and tendons	Very prominent	Fairly prominent	Well covered
Physical Subtotal	_____	_____	_____

FITNESS PROFILE

	WINTER/VATA	SUMMER/PITTA	SPRING/KAPHA
Exercise tolerance	Low	Medium	High
Endurance	Fair	Good	Excellent
Strength	Fair	Better than average	Excellent
Speed	Very good	Good	Not so fast
Competition	Don't like competitive pressure	Driven competitor	Deals easily with competitive pressure
Walking speed	Fast	Average	Slow and steady
Muscle tone	Lean, low body fat	Medium, with good definition	Brawny/bulky, with higher fat percentage
Body size	Small frame, lean or long	Medium frame	Large frame, fleshy
Reaction time	Quick	Average	Slow
Fitness Subtotal	_____	_____	_____

DOSHA GRAND TOTALS

	WINTER/VATA	SUMMER/PITTA	SPRING/KAPHA
Mental			
Behavioral			
Emotional			
Physical			
Fitness			
GRAND TOTALS	_____	_____	_____

Circle your overall highest score and your highest score for the Fitness Profile. If they are the same, choose activities from the one. If they are different, try to combine exercises from both.

- VATA: focus on centering activities such as yoga, walking, biking, martial arts, tai chi, and dancing
- PITTA: focus on weight training, circuit training, biking, hiking, swimming, tennis, mountain climbing, and skiing
- KAPHA: focus on aerobic activity that works up a good sweat, such as BRISK walking, jogging, running, aerobics, spinning, dancing, circuit training, and rowing

Please keep your workout time to one hour or less per day.

My Exercise Plan for next week will be:

Activity	Day/Time/Duration	Place
REST DAY		

Cognitive Health

Dance

In 2008, *Scientific American* released an article from a Columbia University neuroscientist who suggested that synchronizing music and movement created a "pleasure double play." Music stimulates the brain's reward centers, while dance activates its sensory and motor circuits.

PET scans have confirmed that several regions of the brain are active while dancing, specifically the motor cortex, the somatosensory cortex and the basal ganglia. A 2003 study in the *New England Journal of Medicine* by researchers at the Albert Einstein College of Medicine reported that dance lowers dementia risk. Dance has also been found to be therapeutic for patients with Parkinson's disease. According to the Parkinson's Disease Foundation, the primary motor symptoms of Parkinson's disease include bradykinesia (slowed movement), stiffness of the limbs and trunk, tremors, and impaired balance and coordination. These are the symptoms that dance may help alleviate. Tai chi is a Chinese martial art once used for self-defense but is now performed by many as exercise and is considered to be a more ritualized, structured form of dance. Dance and tai chi not only improve cognitive function but also strength, balance, flexibility, and coordination.

The great thing about dance is you can do it in the privacy of your own home. Turn on some music and dance! If you want to maximize how dance can improve cognitive function, find specific dances on YouTube and learn the moves or find a local dance or tai chi class. Classes are great because you also meet new people and share laughter! And laughter makes everything better!

CHAPTER E PREP

1. Continue Chapter A's affirmation until you believe it.
   I fully love and accept you just as you are right now.
2. Begin Chapter E's affirmation (still to be done looking only at your eyes, repeating seven times, morning and night).
   I am a person of great worth.
3. If cravings are still a struggle, continue to experiment with the cravings segment.
4. Foam roll and do the corrective exercises as a warmup for each workout day this. And continue to foam roll daily.
5. Continue practicing deep breathing.
6. If sleep is still an issue, continue to monitor your sleep quality and experiment with the tools provided until you find something that works. If you have found something, record it here_____.
7. Work your Circle of Life action steps and record your progress below:

   _____
   _____
   _____

8. Recognize and handle signs of distress as they pop up this week. Record below.

   _____
   _____
   _____

9. Recognize and address any disordered eating patterns as they surface this week and record below. If you feel you have an actual eating disorder, make an appointment with a professional counselor who deals with eating disorders.

_____

_____

_____

CHAPTER E

Emotional Health

Emotional Tune-up

Check out www.rhondahuff.com for the video lesson, "Chapter E"

In the Chapter A Prep we discussed that emotions are neutral and are simply cues for us to pay attention. I hope you have begun to pay attention to your emotions without judgment. It may have been confusing, frustrating, and constantly changing. And that is OK. When dealing with our emotions, it is rarely a simple or pain-free process. The important thing is to keep at it! The easy thing to do is give up, and while that is an option, it is a very limiting one. If you want growth, keep exploring.

Try this exercise. I want you to choose an emotion that seems to keep resurfacing no matter what you do. You may have a very difficult time looking at this emotion as neutral because it may feel like it has a life beyond your control.

The emotion I am dealing with is

_____

_____

_____

It causes me to behave this way

_____

_____

_____

Once you have named the emotion and the behavior, we want to determine the *positive intention* behind both. This is a precept of Neuro-Linguistic Programming (think author and life coach, Tony Robbins). Every emotion or behavior we have has a purpose. And no matter how horribly this emotion may make us feel or behave, its purpose is either now or was at some time in the past actually positive. Another way to look at this is that any behavior or thought is doing something for us. It is fueling us in some way. It is fulfilling a psychological need, and we may not even realize it. This may seem strange, but it is oh so exciting! Let's dig right in.

When I am feeling the emotion I listed above and I am behaving as I listed above, I am needing/desiring/wanting

_____

_____

_____

Now that you know the positive intention behind the emotion, it is time to have a discussion with the other parts of your psyche. Yes, I want you to talk to yourself. And I want you to write about the discussion.

Here is an example of what I am asking you to do:

Psyche Part 1: When I feel inadequate I become *easily offended when my boss questions my actions.* I want to feel like *I am good enough.* Therefore, I recognize that the positive intention behind feeling inadequate and getting offended is actually the desire to feel like I am good enough.

Psyche Part 2: What is preventing you from feeling good enough?

Psyche Part 1: Because most of the time when I try something new, I fail. And when my boss questions me, it is a reminder of that. Therefore, I am not good enough.

Psyche Part 2: So, you feel inadequate when you are trying something new?

Psyche Part 1: Yes.

Psyche Part 2: Do you fail every single time?

Psyche Part 1: No. But most of the time.

Psyche Part 2: What happened during the occasions that you succeeded?

Psyche Part 1: Once, I got a promotion.

Psyche Part 2: And how did that change your life?

Psyche Part 1: I had to move to a new location, my wife didn't want to go and hated it. We ended up divorced.

Do you see what happened here? Can you see that the feeling of inadequacy actually had more to do with the fear of *SUCCESS* than the need to be good enough? We do this all the time to ourselves. What is the stubborn emotion that keeps you in bondage really trying to do for you? It may be something that you haven't even considered.

We self-sabotage many times based on something that is locked away in our subconscious and may have happened many years ago. So, the answer isn't always simple, but it is always there. In the Chapter E video I will be walking you through a technique that will help you uncover the key to your specific emotion. If you have figured it out already by following the example, that's great! Watch the video anyway because you can talk yourself through these steps in the future.

Record your own conversation with yourself below. There may be more than two parts of yourself that you must engage. Also, this work is usually within your subconscious awareness. Trying to discuss these things with your conscious mind will get you nowhere. So, during this conversation, get into a quiet and relaxed state (I show you how to do this on the video). The subconscious mind is a million times more powerful than the conscious mind and responsible for 94 to 99 percent of all decisions we make. TRUE and LASTING change must happen in the subconscious!

My Conversation with Myself:

_____

_____

_____

Nutritional Health

Eliminations

In Chapter B I asked you to "Build a Better Plan." Now is the time to look back at your own personal observation of foods that may be causing you problems. Compare your list with the list below. Are you having problems with known problematic foods? If so, you are in good company.

Common Problematic Foods:	Possible Reasons Why
Beef, conventionally raised	The GMO grains they are fed, hormones, antibiotics
Coffee	Caffeine, pesticides
Corn (which is a grain, not a vegetable)	Lectins, glyphosate/GMO
Corn oil, sunflower oil, soybean oil	Lectins, glyphosate/GMO
Dairy	Hormones (the cows have to be pregnant to produce milk so eventhough RSBT isn't added, there are still plenty of hormones that can wreak havoc on your body), lactose, casein A1
Eggs	The protein in the egg or something the chicken ate
Gluten grains: barley, rye, spelt, wheat	Gluten, glyphosate/GMO
Legumes: beans, peas, soybeans, lentils, etc.	Lectins, phytic acid
Milk chocolate	Milk, wheat
Nightshades: white potatoes, peppers, eggplant gogi berries, tomatoes	Lectins and the neurotoxin, solanine
Peanuts and cashews	Lectins
Pork	Alpha-galactose, albumin allergy
Processed meats	Nitrates, nitrites, preservatives, glutamates
Quinoa	Lectins
Shellfish	Protein
Soy	Lectins, glyphosate/GMO
Squashes	Lectins, sugar
Tea	Caffeine, tannins, catechins, oils
White (table) sugar	Fructose, sucrose, something in the refining process

If you are reacting negatively to any of the above foods, begin eliminating them. It doesn't mean you can never have them again, it just means you need to allow your digestive tract time to rest and heal.

If you aren't sure if something is a problem, take it out of your plan for seven days. On the eighth day, eat it and pay attention to what your body tells you. Check in with your emotions, your brain, and your body.

If the Lone Star tick has bitten you, it can create an allergy to beef and pork.

If you are allergic to cats, you also may be allergic to pork.

If you are primarily responding to foods containing lectins and/or phytic acid, it may be the way you are preparing them. Here are the best and safest preparation methods.

- Soak legumes for at least twelve hours and then rinse them thoroughly before cooking.
- Sprout legumes by soaking them between twelve and twenty-four hours, straining them and then leaving them out to sprout. Sprouting also can boost the amount of beneficial nutrients.
- Ferment legumes. This typically involves combining seeds with yeast and an acid to create healthy bacteria that can then help you break them down. If you have Parkinson's disease, or a family history of Parkinson's disease, you should be careful not to eat too many fermented foods.

Physical Health

Exercise

In Chapter D you discovered your Dosha Exercise Type(s). For the next six weeks, commit to the type(s) of exercise your body may be telling you that you need. If you already have a workout plan that you do consistently and are happy with, you may continue with that. However, if you want to mix it up for six weeks, the body loves variety and you may be surprised how much you enjoy it!

My exercise plan for the next six weeks will be:

WEEK 1

Activity	Day/Time/Duration	Place

REST DAY		

WEEK 2

Activity	Day/Time/Duration	Place
REST DAY		

WEEK 3

Activity	Day/Time/Duration	Place
REST DAY		

WEEK 4

Activity	Day/Time/Duration	Place
REST DAY		

WEEK 5

Activity	Day/Time/Duration	Place
REST DAY		

WEEK 6

Activity	Day/Time/Duration	Place
REST DAY		

The self-assessment below is CRUCIAL so please pay attention to these areas. It will be used to determine your next workout program.

After six weeks, these are the changes I have noticed. Place a check by the ones that apply to you.

Body composition

_____I have improved muscularity and/or muscle tone

_____I have lost bodyfat

_____I have lost inches—overall this many_____

_____My clothes fit better OR I have lost _____ size(s)

Energy

_____I have more energy

_____I feel younger

_____I am sleeping better

Injuries

_____ I did not sustain injuries during the six weeks

_____ Old injuries do not flare up as often as before

Cardiovascular/pulmonary

_____ I feel less winded upon exertion

_____ I notice an ability to "keep up" with my kids/grandkids/friends better than before

_____ I notice less swelling/puffiness in my body than before

_____ My blood pressure is better

Strength

_____ Daily activities seem easier than before

_____ Stairs are easier than before

_____ I do feel stronger

Mental/emotional

_____ I am able to handle stress more easily

_____ I feel calmer

_____ My moods are more stable

_____ I feel happier

_____ My mind is clearer. "The fog has lifted."

_____ I found the workouts enjoyable

Cognitive Health

Evaluating Core Beliefs

For this chapter's cognitive health segment, I am simply going to make you think. We will be using the Circle of Life from Chapter C so have that handy. We will also use this chapter's _Emotional Tune-up_.

Core beliefs are defined as fundamental, inflexible, absolute, and generalized beliefs that people hold about themselves, others, the world, and/or the future.

According to Cognitive Behavioral Therapy, "when a core belief is inaccurate, unhelpful, and/or judgmental (e.g., 'I am worthless'), it has a profound effect on a person's self-concept, sense of self-efficacy, and continued vulnerability to mood disturbance. Core beliefs typically center around themes of lovability (e.g., 'I am undesirable'), adequacy ('I am incompetent'), and/or helplessness (e.g., 'I am trapped')."

Using a combination of Cognitive Behavioral Therapy's Downward Arrow Technique, Neuro-Linguistic Programming Techniques, and Primary Foods© Analysis, you will begin to unravel the mysteries of your own beliefs. You will ask yourself questions such as: What are my core beliefs? Where did they come from? Are they relevant and helpful to my life now? Do I need to change them?

Look at your Circle of Life elements. You are working on action steps to improve your satisfaction level in your lowest three scores. How is that going? Do you see some movement in the right direction or are you stuck? If you are stuck, it may be because your core belief about that area is preventing it. So, let's get curious and explore that.

Follow the example below. Your grids are after the example. Complete the grids for the lowest three Circle of Life elements. You may need more or less room than what is provided. That's OK. Modify it as needed. The purpose is to find the core belief and evaluate it.

We will work on changing these core beliefs later in the program. Right now, I want you to get clear about the belief, where it came from, its limitations on your life, and if you are ready and willing to change it.

Example:

#12
Relationships
I am working on improving my relationship with my coworkers.
What Core Belief may be preventing this from happening?
I feel like I am not as good as my coworkers.
Where did that belief come from?
My mom always told me there would always be someone better than I am.
What does it mean that someone will always be better than you?
It means that I am inferior and I will never be the best.
What will it mean if you are never the best?
It will mean that I just have to "stay in my place."
What will it mean to you if you decide to "stay in your place?"
It will mean that I don't develop relationships with my co-workers. I will just work and go home.
What will it mean to your coworkers if you decide to "stay in your place?"
My coworkers will never really know me or my abilities.
What will it mean to you if your coworkers never know you or your abilities?
They won't know that I have good ideas that can make the company better and make all of us more money.
What would company growth and more money mean to your coworkers?
It would probably make them happy.

So by developing relationships with your coworkers you would be happier and they would be happier?
Yes, I think so.

MODIFY CORE BELIEF

#12

What Core Belief may be preventing this from happening?

Where did that belief come from?

What does it mean that _____?

What will it mean if _____?

What will it mean to you if _____?

What will it mean to others if you _____?

What will it mean to you if _____?

What would conquering this mean to others?

What would conquering this mean to you?

MODIFY CORE BELIEF

#11

What Core Belief may be preventing this from happening?

Where did that belief come from?

What does it mean that _____?

What will it mean if _____?

What will it mean to you if _____?
What will it mean to others if you _____?
What will it mean to you if _____?
What would conquering this mean to others?
What would conquering this mean to you?
MODIFY CORE BELIEF

#10
What Core Belief may be preventing this from happening?
Where did that belief come from?
What does it mean that _____?
What will it mean if _____?
What will it mean to you if _____?
What will it mean to others if you _____?
What will it mean to you if _____?
What would conquering this mean to others?
What would conquering this mean to you?
MODIFY CORE BELIEF

CHAPTER F PREP

1. Continue Chapter A's affirmation until you believe it.
   I fully love and accept you just as you are right now.
2. Begin Chapter F's affirmation (still to be done looking only at your eyes, repeating seven times, morning and night).
   I speak with integrity and ask for what I need.
3. If cravings are still a struggle, ask yourself if you are truly using the techniques given, especially eating more greens. What tweaks can you make to allow these techniques to work? Record here:

   _____
   _____
   _____

4. Foam roll and do the corrective exercises as a warmup for each workout day this week. And continue to foam roll daily. Remember to record your workouts.
5. Continue practicing deep breathing.
6. If sleep is still an issue, continue to monitor your sleep quality and experiment with the tools provided until you find something that works. If you found something last week, record it here_____.
7. Continue getting curious about the relationship between your Circle of Life elements and your Core Beliefs. Dig deep!

8. Recognize and handle distress as it pops up this week. Record below.

   _____

   _____

   _____

9. How are your eating patterns going? Are you at four hours between meals and a twelve-hour fast between dinner and breakfast? (Remember if you are diabetic, you are to clear all modifications with your doctor.)

CHAPTER F

Emotional Health

Four Agreements

Check out www.rhondahuff.com for the video lesson, "Chapter F"

After reading *The Four Agreements: A Practical Guide to Personal Freedom* by author Don Miguel Ruiz, something in my mind-set shifted. I was liberated from years of feeling like I was always letting someone down. It seemed that no matter how hard I tried, nothing was good enough. *The Four Agreements* was instrumental in helping me see that I was living in the presupposition of someone else's reality. You may be wondering what that even means. It means that most days I would make decisions based on what I thought someone else would think. Would that person agree or disagree? Would that person be pleased or displeased? Could I live with the repercussions of either? The only person who truly knows your mind, heart, and intentions is God Himself. I believe that often WE don't even know our true mind, heart, or intentions. We are not gods. Many belief systems claim we can become enlightened to the point of being a god. I completely disagree with this and here's why: No matter how enlightened someone becomes, they do not know the thoughts of others. We can become better at empathy to the point of almost feeling what others feel. But we will never be able to know what others think or intend. Making assumptions about the intentions of others is one sure way to become a miserable person. No matter how well we know someone, we do not know his or her intentions. Only God can do that.

I am so excited to share the Four Agreements with you! I will share more about my experience with *The Four Agreements* on the Chapter F video.

The Four Agreements are:

1. **Be impeccable with your word:** Speak with integrity. Say only what you mean. Be clear about what you need. Avoid using words to speak against yourself or to gossip about others. Use the power of your words in the direction of truth and love.

2. **Don't take anything personally:** Nothing others do is because of you. What others say and do is a projection of their own reality, their own dream. When you are immune to the opinions and actions of others, you won't be the victim of needless suffering. This is true in the negative and the positive. Once you realize that someone's POSITIVE opinion of you is merely a reflection of his or her own reality and has little to do with you, it will make it easier to let go of the negative as well.

3. **Don't make assumptions:** Find the courage to ask questions and to express what you really want. Communicate with others clearly to avoid misunderstandings, sadness and drama. I remember learning at a young age that to "assume" would make an "ass" out of "u" and "me."

4. **Always do your best:** Your best is going to change from day to day, and perhaps, from moment to moment. Your best will be different when you are healthy as opposed to sick, calm as opposed to stressed, happy as opposed to sad. Under any circumstance, simply do your best, and you will avoid self-judgment, self-abuse, and regret. Stop comparing your accomplishments to what they were twenty years ago. Your best now is different from your best then. Just live one day at a time, knowing that you are doing the best you can with what you have right now at this very moment.

Which agreements resonate the most with you? Why?

_____

_____

_____

How will you implement these principles into your daily life?

_____

_____

_____

Nutritional Health

FOOD©

Several years ago, I came up with a simple acronym to remind people to just eat real food. I have expanded this to explain the why behind each concept.

F ree of anti-nutrients

O rganic when possible

O riginal in form

D ense in nutrients

F is for Free of Anti-nutrients

Anti-nutrients are often the same thing as *unpronounceables*. The general rule of thumb is: "If you can't pronounce it, don't eat it. And even if you can pronounce it, if it has more than five ingredients, put it back."

Manufacturing companies get very creative in order to continue to use products that we are continually learning are not healthy. Below is a list of just a few of the anti-nutrients that surround us every day.

Trans Fats	
cottonseed oil	hydrogenated oils (of any kind)
lard	mono-diglycerides
monoglycinate	partially hydrogenated oil (of any kind)
shortening	interesterified oils

Glutamtes (MSG)	
calcium caseinate	autolyzed yeast
gelatin	corn oil
glutamic acid	glutamate

hydrolyzed protein (wheat, milk, oat, soy, whey, vegetable, plant)	hydrolyzed corn gluten
monosodium glutamate	monopotassium glutamate
"natural flavoring"	plant protein extract
sodium caseinate	natrium glutamate
"spices"	soy protein isolate
yeast extract	textured protein (TVP—texturized vegetable protein)
yeast nutrient	yeast food

Preservatives	
(1, 1 dimethylethyl)-4-methoxy	anisole
antioxyne b	antrancine 12
benzic acid	butylated hydroxyanisole (bha)
butylated hydroxytoluene (bht)	butylhydroxyanisole
embanox	nepantiox 1-f
olestra	phenol
potassium bromate	propyl gallate
sodium benzoate	sodium bisulfate
sodium chloride (salt)	sodium dioxide
sodium nitrate	sodium nitrite
sustane 1-f	tenox bha
tert-butyl hydrox	tert-butyl-4-methoxy

Artificial colors	
allura red AC (E129)	blue 1 and 2
carmoisine (E122)	green 3
ponceau 4R (E124)	quinoline yellow (E104)
red 3	sunset yellow (E110)
tartrazine (E102)	yellow 6

Sweeteners	
acesulfame K (sunett)	Alitame
aspartame (AminoSweet, NutraSweet, Equal)	Cyclamate

Erythritol (Truvia)—powerful insecticide	high fructose corn syrup
(HFCS-90, HFCS-55, and HFCS-42)	neotame
saccharin (Sweet 'n Low)	sucralose (Splenda)
white sugar	

O is for Organic when Possible

Simply stated, organic produce is grown without the use of pesticides, synthetic fertilizers, sewage sludge, genetically modified organisms, or ionizing radiation. Animals that produce meat, poultry, eggs, and dairy products do not take antibiotics or growth hormones.

Check the bar code on your produce. A 5-digit code that starts with the number "9" indicates the produce is organic.

I know it is hard to always buy organic, especially if you are feeding a large family. Use this chart provided by ewg.org to help you make better choices.

Always buy organic	**OK to buy conventional**
apples	asparagus
celery	avocados
cherry tomatoes	cabbage
collards	cantaloupe
cucumbers	cauliflower
grapes	eggplant
hot peppers	grapefruit
kale	kiwi
nectarines	mangoes
peaches	onions
potatoes	papayas
snap peas	pineapples
spinach	sweet corn
strawberries	sweet peas
sweet bell peppers	sweet potatoes

O is for Original in Form

Okay, let me just get this out of the way now. One of my biggest pet peeves is food that has shapes. The one I fed my kids (before I knew better) was chicken nuggets that are shaped like dinosaurs. If you are eating a chicken breast, it should look like a chicken breast. And it shouldn't be huge. Chickens in their natural, non-steroid, non-saline world are quite small. Choose grass-fed meats, free-range poultry, and wild-caught fish.

D is for Dense in Nutrients

Eat the rainbow! Eating a colorful variety of vegetables and fruits ensures you will get a full spectrum of nutrients. Here is a list of just the basics of what the color of the produce can tell you.

Red = Lycopene. Lycopene is a powerful antioxidant that can help reduce the risk of cancer and protect the heart.

Orange/Yellow = Carotenoids. Betacarotene is converted to vitamin A, which helps maintain healthy mucous membranes and healthy eyes. Lutein has been found to prevent cataracts and age-related macular degeneration. Other carotenoids improve the immune system and prevent cancer and heart disease.

Green = Phytochemicals, including chlorophyll as well as isothiocyanates, which have anti-cancer properties and protects against birth defects.

Blue/Purple = Anthocyanins. Anthocyanins has antioxidant properties that protect cells from damage, improves memory, promotes healthy aging, and can help reduce the risk of cancer, stroke and heart disease.

Brown/White = Anthoxanthins. Anthoxanthins are phytochemicals such as allicin (found in garlic), which is known for its antiviral, antibacterial, and anti-inflammatory properties. Anthoxanthins also lower cholesterol and blood pressure, reduces the risk of stomach cancer, and reduces the risk of heart disease.

Therefore, healthy eating means eating a variety of foods that give you the nutrients you need to maintain your health, feel well, and have energy.

- Replace "Will this make me gain or lose *weight*?" with "Will this make me gain or lose *health*?"
- Eat the rainbow everyday
- If your great-great-great grandmother would recognize it, chances are so will your body (vegetables, fruits, legumes, beans, seeds, nuts, fish, meat)
- Stop eating when you are about four-fifths full
- *"Eat food, not too much, mostly plants."* (Michael Pollan, author, journalist, activist)

Physical Health

Floss and Scrape
Floss

How often do you floss? Flossing is an important step in staying healthy! Many people state that they don't like to floss because it causes their teeth to bleed. That is an even bigger reason to floss. Healthy gums do NOT bleed when flossed. Dentists say they can go in between healthy gums with a dental instrument and they won't bleed.

Unhealthy gums bleed. The blood is sent to your gums to fight off the infection and bacteria. The problem is that your body senses your tooth as the infection and tries to get rid of your tooth (hence bone loss around the tooth and eventual tooth loss if not treated). Flossing also does about 40 percent of the work required for healthy gums by removing the sticky bacteria (plaque) from the tooth's surface. Brushing alone misses at least two of the five surfaces of the teeth. Even minor gum disease can also ruin the youthful appearance of your smile by eating away at gums and teeth.

Some research has shown a link between unhealthy gums and disease. Though this may still be true, most medical professionals are now saying the true underlying link to all disease is inflammation and that curbing inflammation through proper nutrition and lifestyle can prevent many diseases, including periodontal disease.

So, grab that floss! You will look younger, feel better, and have better breath!

Scrape

The tongue cleaner, an inexpensive yet transformative utensil, is a simple, thin piece of stainless steel. (Don't use plastic that harbors germs). It consists of a blunted edge that removes plaque and build-up from the surface of the tongue. Dentists in America are recommending the tongue cleaner more and more because it helps to fight cavities by removing bacteria from the mouth. The tongue cleaner also prevents bad breath, especially for people who eat a lot of dairy and build up mucus in the mouth, nose, and throat.

The tongue cleaner comes from the tradition of Ayurveda, which asserts that people who use one are better at public speaking, express themselves more thoughtfully, and speak more sincerely and authoritatively. Some people ask if the same effect can be gained by brushing the tongue with a stiff toothbrush. Brushing the tongue moves stuff around and is helpful, but a tongue cleaner is more effective as it clears out the deep deposits and keeps the area cleaner, stimulated and alive.

Also, **cravings** can be reduced by cleaning the tongue of leftover food. When your mouth can still taste the food, you may experience cravings for previously eaten foods. A tongue cleaner reverses the process of desensitizing your taste buds, which has happened to everyone to a greater or lesser extent. It allows you to taste more subtle flavors in food so that you can eat vegetables, fruits and whole grains with greater joy. When old residue is removed from the tongue, you will be better able to taste your food and won't need to eat as much since you will have gained greater satisfaction from your meal.

And finally, a big advantage is that it enhances kissing because it makes the tongue more sweet, fresh and sensitive. If you are in a relationship, we invite you to check this out with your partner. Make an agreement to scrape twice a day for one week and notice the difference.

Directions:
- Apply a few quick strokes, two to three times a day, or after brushing your teeth.
- Use the rounded cleaning edge to scrape gently down the tongue several times, while applying slight pressure.
- Rinse under running water and gently scrape again until no white residue is left.
- There should be no pain or gagging involved whatsoever. If you feel any discomfort, you are scraping too hard or starting too far back on the tongue.
- And if you are wondering what those bumps are at the back of your tongue, they are your salivary glands and they are supposed to be there. If you found them you've gone too far.

Cognitive Health

Fifteen Fun Facts About Your Brain
1. When our eyes receive images, they are upside-down. Our brain automatically adjusts them so that we see images right side up.
2. An adult brain weighs about three pounds.
3. It is the fattest organ in the body, with the solid tissue comprised of 60 percent fat.
4. It is a myth that humans only use 10 percent of our brain. We actually use all of it. We're even using more than 10 percent when we sleep.

5. Cholesterol is key for learning and memory.
6. Our fastest neurons pass along information at about 250 mph.
7. The solid tissue in the brain may be 60 percent fat, but overall the brain is 75 percent water. This means dehydration can be a huge problem.
8. The brain can't feel pain. It interprets pain signals sent to it, but it does not feel pain. That's why surgeons can operate on the brain while the patient is awake.
9. A brain freeze is really a sphenopalatine ganglioneuralgia. It happens when you eat or drink something that's cold. It is believed to result from a nerve response causing rapid constriction and swelling of blood vessels that refers pain from the roof of the mouth to the head.
10. Your brain uses 20 percent of the oxygen and blood in your body.
11. Dreaming requires more brain activity than anything we do while awake!
12. Music improves brain organization.
13. Every time you recall a memory or have a new thought, you create a new neuronal connection.
14. The average person has 70,000 thoughts per day.
15. There are enough blood vessels in your brain to wrap around the earth four times.

CHAPTER G PREP

1. Continue Chapter A's affirmation until you believe it.
   I fully love and accept you just as you are right now.
2. Begin Chapter G's affirmation (still to be done looking only at your eyes, repeating seven times, morning and night).
   I am grateful and blessed.
3. If cravings are still a struggle, ask yourself if you are truly using the techniques given, especially eating more greens. What tweaks can you make to allow these techniques to work? Record here:

   _____

   _____

   _____

4. Foam roll and do the corrective exercises as a warmup for each workout day this week. And continue to foam roll daily. Remember to record your workouts.
5. Continue practicing deep breathing.
6. If sleep is still an issue, continue to monitor your sleep quality and experiment with the tools provided until you find something that works. If you found something, record it here.

   _____

   _____

   _____

7. Continue getting curious about the relationship between your Circle of Life elements and your Core Beliefs. Dig deep.

8. Recognize and handle distress as it pops up this week. Record below.

_____

_____

_____

9. How are your eating patterns going? Are you at four hours between meals and a twelve-hour fast between dinner and breakfast? (Remember if you are diabetic, you are to clear all modifications with your doctor.)

10. Remember the Four Agreements. Which one has been a challenge this week? Explore why.

11. Use the FOOD© principle as you grocery shop and prepare meals.

CHAPTER G

Emotional Health

Grief's Positive Purpose—the Goodbye Exercise

University of Houston research professor Dr. Brené Brown is one of my favorite authors. Back in December 2015, I read her book, *Rising Strong*. She states in the book that she had been dealing with the issue of forgiveness for ten years. Brown is a social scientist and a grounded-theory researcher so she only publishes what she can scientifically prove. When dealing with forgiveness she couldn't find a meaningful pattern that didn't have outliers, which in the grounded-theory approach isn't allowed. She goes on to share that one day while at church her pastor spoke on forgiveness. Her pastor spoke what many of you have probably heard from your own pews, "In order for forgiveness to happen, something has to die. If you make a choice to forgive, you have to face into pain. You simply have to hurt."

Brown had her answer. She realized in that moment that forgiveness is so difficult because it involves death and grief. Her research before had been looking at patterns in people extending forgiveness and love, but not in people experiencing grief. She puts it beautifully,

> *"Given the dark fears we feel when we experience loss, nothing is more generous and loving than the willingness to embrace grief in order to forgive. To be forgiven is to be loved."*

As I read further, I was brought to my knees.

"The death or ending that forgiveness necessitates comes in many shapes and forms. We may need to bury our expectations or dreams…"

My dream! Oh, my dream! I sobbed uncontrollably as the issue of forgiving my ex-husband came flooding to the forefront of my thoughts. My biggest dream since July of 2011 was that I would be reconciled to my husband of 28 years. Our marriage was toxic. He was angry and violent, and I was stubborn and withdrawn. The more he tried to control and intimidate me, the more withdrawn and stubborn I became. And the more withdrawn and stubborn I became, the more angry and violent he became. It was a vicious cycle. One that led me to decide that I just couldn't live that way anymore. I remember telling my best friend, "Life is too LONG to live like this."

But one thing was certain, I truly did love my husband and I longed for his relationship with me and with our children to be what it was supposed to be, not what it was. I fully trusted that God would change things for us, that we would one day be a family again.

It was no coincidence that I was reading Brown's book two weeks before my ex-husband was getting remarried. When I learned of his engagement in January 2015, I sank into a deep depression. Yet I still held out hope that he would choose to put our family back together. Looking back at last year, it was a full year of "episodes." One moment I was fine and rationally thinking about the fact that things would have never been better between us, and that I emotionally couldn't live like I was living before. The next I was in the pit wallowing in the deepest ache I have ever felt, knowing that we wouldn't be together as our grandbabies were born, or as birthdays were celebrated, or as weddings were planned. For a couple of weeks after moving back to Virginia in July, I didn't even want to get out of bed. I had left my safe place, my hiding place in New York City and now was face to face with the past. I wasn't prepared for the emotional turmoil I felt.

I had been trying to forgive him for years at this point. I tried praying, I tried meditating, I tried visualizing. I even tried guilting myself into forgiveness by reminding myself that Christ had forgiven me. That didn't work either. Nothing did! I just couldn't forgive him. And I really didn't know why. I had never had a problem forgiving people before. And my lack of forgiveness had begun to turn into hatred. A feeling that was completely foreign to me. I don't think I have ever HATED anything in my life, especially not people. But here I was, feeling hatred toward a man I once loved with all my heart.

But Brown's words gave me freedom. You see, one thing that many people had shared with me was that to forgive him I had to die to self. People, I was broken! I already felt dead. How does one die to self when there isn't any perceivable "self" left to die? I remember thinking to myself, "If anymore of me dies, there will be nothing left."

But Brown said SOMETHING had to die. She didn't say I had to die. And I knew right away it was my dream that had to die. The dream that someday my family would be back together. It was time for a funeral. It was time to say goodbye to that dream.

What have you boxed up and set aside that may be preventing you from living a full and rewarding life? Take some time to think about the person or people you may need to forgive. You may need to forgive yourself. Is it time for a funeral? Is it time to grieve? It's hard, horrible, actually. But it is necessary.

Love yourself enough to let go.

Record your thoughts below. If necessary, write a eulogy for what needs to die (I did). And then burn it or bury it. Give yourself permission to grieve.

_____

_____

_____

Nutritional Health

Gut Health

"Heal the gut and you heal yourself."
—**Dr. Gerard E. Mullin, MD**, author and associate professor
of medicine at Johns Hopkins University Hospital.

Poor gut health has been implicated in:

- Inflammatory conditions such as gout, Irritable Bowel Syndrome, arthritis, asthma, colitis, diverticulitis, and Parkinson's disease.
- Auto-immune diseases such as diabetes, Epstein-Barr, celiac, Hashimoto's thyroiditis, interstitial cystitis, juvenile diabetes, juvenile arthritis, lyme

disease, multiple sclerosis, psoriasis, Raynaud's phenomenon, sarcoidosis, and rheumatoid arthritis

- Conditions that are related to both inflammation and auto-immunity such as lupus, Crohn's, endometriosis, and fibromyalgia (research shows that up to 78 percent of people with fibromyalgia have Small Intestinal Bacterial Overgrowth, also known as SIBO)
- Other conditions are also implicated, including allergies, autism, ADD, ADHD, obsessive-compulsive disorder, and dyslexia, just to name a few.

Common causes of poor gut health:

- Medical therapies such as radiation or chemotherapy
- Medications, especially antibiotics and NSAIDs
- Poor diet: alcohol, sugar, preservatives, processed foods, over-eating, inadequate fiber intake, etc.
- Poor gut motility
- Stress (stress hormones may encourage bad bacterial growth)
- Too much animal-based protein, especially highly processed ones like lunch meats

On the flip side, a good microbiome supports proper weight (studies show that a fecal transplant from an obese person to a thin person causes instant weight gain), nutritional absorption, genetic expression, proper manufacturing of vitamins B3, B5, B6, B12, K, folate, and biotin, proper gut function/protection, and energy availability. Children who are delivered vaginally have a gut flora that contains more pathogen-protecting bacteria than children who are delivered via C-section.

Let's focus on the positives of the gut and get the gut in gear! I recently attended a medical conference where thet issue of gut dysbiosis (microbial imbalance) was discussed at length. Helen Messier, MD, PhD, shared that the skin hosts a trillion resident bacteria, the mouth hosts 10 billion, and the gut hosts 100 trillion (two to five pounds of your bodyweight is gut bacteria)

A healthy gut barrier depends on:

- Balanced intestinal bacteria (that two to five pounds I just mentioned)
- An intact mucosa (the gut lining replaces itself every three to seven days)
- A healthy immune system (70 percent of our immune system cells live in or around the gut)

There are a number of ways you can have your gut assessed:

- Stool Testing
  - Microscopy
  - EIA Antigen Testing
  - Culture / PCR
  - Metabolites
- Breath Testing
- Urinary Organic Acid Testing

You can take probiotics as a supplement, which will increase the good bacteria as long as you keep taking it. Probiotics are good bacteria that assist the health of your digestive system by controlling the growth of harmful bacteria. They enhance the microbial balance, restoring intestinal permeability and gut microecology. Consult with a Functional Medicine Physician to find out the best dosage and type for you.

The best option is to improve the gut flora permanently through nutrition.

Probiotic-rich foods: one to two servings daily	
Buttermilk	Fermented vegetables
Kefir	Kimchi
Kombucha	Miso
Natto	Oats
Pulke	Quinoa
Raw pickles	Raw vinegars
Root and ginger beers	Sauerkraut
Tempeh	Wine (4 oz)
Yogurt	

Prebiotics are complex carbohydrates that cannot be digested by the human body. Prebiotics become food for probiotics.

Prebiotic-rich foods: two to three servings daily	
Asparagus	Bananas
Berries	Bran
Burdock root	Chicory

Chinese chives	Cottage cheese
Dandelion greens	Eggplant
Garlic	Green tea
Honey	Jerusalem artichokes
Kefir	Leeks
Legumes	Onions
Peas	Psyllium
Rye	Yogurt

Work on adding probiotic-rich and prebiotic-rich foods into your daily nutrition plan.

Please note that you may actually feel worse before you feel better since bacteria will release toxins. You may feel a bit more gassy or bloated in the beginning. It should settle down within a few days. Immune-compromised individuals can develop infections from probiotic microbes so be cautious if you are taking immunosuppressive drugs, if you have AIDS, if you are receiving radiation or chemotherapy, or if you are in the hospital. Consult your physician for specifics.

Physical Health

Glutes

Check out www.rhondahuff.com for the video lesson, "Chapter G"

We are taking a little walk back to Chapter C, *Correctives*. During our video we mentioned that often people simply do not engage the glutes in a way that provides protection for the knee, low back, hamstrings, and groin and creates movement efficiency.

The glutes are the largest and strongest muscles in your body. They consist of three muscles: gluteus minimus, medius and maximus. Strengthening the glutes will result in making normal everyday activities, such as standing up, sitting down, lifting objects, and climbing stairs easier. Developing strong glutes also improves athletic performance and decreases the risk of injuries. Strong glutes are also aesthetically pleasing.

Let's add a few glute-specific moves to your workout routine this week.

A couple of your correctives that specifically address glutes are the sit to stands and step-ups. If these are still a challenge, continue doing them. If they have gotten easy and you know you are engaging the glutes optimally, then it is time to move on. You may stop doing those two correctives and add these two moves into your routine. Mastering these two moves will ensure that you have adequate strength and proper form for the bigger glute development moves such as full squats, deadlifts, and kettlebell swings.

The Hip Hinge:
(If needed, you can use a dowel or broomstick. You will see this in the video.)

1. Position yourself about six to twelve inches in front of a wall.
2. Take a shoulder width stance with your feet straight ahead.
3. If using a dowel or broomstick, one hand grasps the dowel at the cervical spine (neck) and the other hand grasps the dowel at the lumbar spine (lower back). Maintain three points of contact with the dowel: the head, the thoracic spine, and the sacrum.
4. Bend forward while sitting back and keeping the chest up remembering to maintain your three points of contact if you are using a dowel or broomstick.
5. Your weight should be in your heels.
6. Repeat ten times.

The Glute Bridge:
1. Lie on your back with your hips flexed at approximately 135 degrees and knees at 90 degrees, with a shoulder-width stance and feet straight ahead. I like to lift my toes off the floor but you can keep yours down if preferred.
2. The girl in the picture has her palms down but I prefer for the palms to be up.
3. Keep your weight in your heels as you thrust your hips up.
4. Keep the lumbar spine in neutral. It is not about how high you can lift your hips, it is more about how well you squeeze your glutes.
5. Hold for a count of two and return to the floor.
6. Repeat ten times.

Cognitive Health

Gratitude
Gratitude is simply the practice of being thankful. It is not fake optimism. It is recognizing that life is hard and yet finding things for which to be grateful anyway. Sometimes we can get so busy with the little annoyances in life that we forget to be

thankful. And it turns out that gratitude is super healthy for your brain! Counting your blessings is proven to flood your brain with reward chemicals, lessen depression and anxiety, regulate the hypothalamus—which controls sleep, hunger, metabolism, and temperature—and make you more resistant to the effects of stress. It helps you fall asleep more easily, awaken more refreshed, trains the prefrontal cortex to retain positive information, and makes you a happier person overall.

This exercise is about focusing on the people, places, experiences, and things for which you are grateful. Every night before bed, record three. It may be hard at first, but I promise it will get easier as you train your brain to watch for and remember the many blessings that occur each and every day.

Night	1	2	3
Sunday			
Monday			
Tuesday			
Wednesday			
Thursday			
Friday			
Saturday			

CHAPTER H PREP

1. Continue Chapter A's affirmation until you believe it.
    I fully love and accept you just as you are right now.
2. Begin Chapter H's affirmation (still to be done looking only at your eyes, repeating seven times, morning and night).
    I am becoming the best version of myself.
3. By now, deep breathing and breath awareness should be a habit. Allow this new habit to continue to improve your mind, body, and health.
4. By now, you have had time to experiment with tactics to aid a proper night's sleep. If sleep is still an issue, ask your doctor to refer you to a sleep specialist for a sleep study.
5. If cravings are still a struggle, ask yourself if you are truly using the techniques given, especially eating more greens. What tweaks can you make to allow these techniques to work? Record here:

    _____

    _____

    _____

6. Foam roll and do the corrective exercises as a warmup for each workout day this week. And continue to foam roll daily. Remember to record your workouts.
7. Check in with your Circle of Life. Have any of the scores improved? Especially the lowest three that you have been working on? Do you have a **new lowest three**? Do any of them need a *Goodbye Exercise* for forgiveness? Record here:

What is now ranked Number 12?

_____

_____

_____

Why am I unhappy with this area of my life?

_____

_____

_____

Here is one action step I will take this week to enhance my happiness in this area:

_____

_____

_____

What is now ranked Number 11?

_____

_____

_____

Why am I unhappy with this area of my life?

_____

_____

_____

Here is one action step I will take this week to enhance my happiness in this area:

_____

_____

_____

What is now ranked Number 10?

_____

_____

_____

Why am I unhappy with this area of my life?

_____

_____

_____

Here is one action step I will take this week to enhance my happiness in this area:

_____

_____

_____

8. Recognize and handle distress as it pops up this week. Record below.

_____

_____

_____

9. How are your eating patterns going? Are you at four hours between meals and a twelve-hour fast between dinner and breakfast? (Remember if you are diabetic, you are to clear all modifications with your doctor.)

10. Remember the Four Agreements

11. Use the FOOD© principle and add prebiotic and probiotic foods into your day.

12. Practice gratitude everyday.

13. Focus on foods that improve your gut health.

CHAPTER H

Emotional Health

Highly Sensitive People

A Highly Sensitive Person (HSP) is someone who processes sensory data exceptionally deeply and thoroughly due to a biological difference in his or her nervous system. This term was first coined by Dr. Elaine N. Aron, author of *The Highly Sensitive Person.*

For HSPs, regular sensory information is processed and analyzed at a deep level, which contributes to creativity, intuition, sensing implications and attention to detail. The drawback is a tendency to become over-stimulated very quickly.

Highly Sensitive People have an uncommonly sensitive nervous system. It is a normal occurrence and a distinct personality trait that affects as many as one out of every five people. It means you are aware of details and facets of your surroundings that others often overlook.

This trait is normal. It is inherited by 15 to 20 percent of the population, and indeed the same percentage is present in all higher animals.

Being an HSP means your nervous system is more sensitive to subtleties. Your sight, hearing and sense of smell are not necessarily keener (although they may be). An HSP brain manages information and reflects on it more intensely.

Being an HSP also means being easily over-stimulated, stressed out and overwhelmed.

This trait is not something newly discovered. It has been mislabeled as shyness (not an inherited trait), introversion (30 percent of HSPs are actually extroverts), inhibitedness, fearfulness and the like. HSPs can be these, but none of these is the fundamental trait they have inherited.

In our culture, being tough and outgoing is the preferred or ideal personality. This cultural bias affects HSPs as much as their trait affects them. You may have grown up hearing, "Don't be so sensitive," making you feel abnormal, when in fact you could do nothing about it. The trait is not a flaw or a syndrome, nor is it a reason to brag. It is an asset you can learn to use and protect.

Take this test to see if you are a Highly Sensitive Person http://hsperson.com/test/highly-sensitive-test/

—*The Highly Sensitive Person: How to Thrive When the World Overwhelms You,* by Elaine N. Aron, PhD. Broadway Books, 1996

Nutritional Health

Hot or Cold?

According to Ayurveda, your Dosha may dictate if you will do better with cooked—steamed, sautéed, or simmered, not fried or over-cooked—or raw foods. Raw foods are thought of as being cold, dry, light, rough, and *Rajasic,* a Sanskrit term that means "activating" or "enervating." Consuming foods with these qualities can strain digestion, particularly in someone who already has weak digestion. For these people, too many raw foods can lead to poor absorption of nutrients, lack of nourishment to our tissues, imbalances in our body, and illness or disease.

Minerals and vitamins in some vegetables and fruits are actually more bioavailable when lightly steamed, sautéed, or simmered at low temperatures. In fact, some foods contain anti-nutrients that actually block nutrient absorption and the cooking process can mitigate many of those. And remember that overcooking foods can reduce their nutrient content and *Prana,* a Sanskrit term meaning vital life-force energy.

There are so many theories out about nutrition. It is very difficult to weed through all the research. Once again what it boils down to is *individualization.* Listen to your body. Stop following your friend's diet and discover your own. If for some reason one day the thought of a salad turns your stomach, then don't eat one. Eat cooked vegetables instead. Your body is smart and knows what it needs. Simply learn to really hear what it is saying to you.

Please consult your Dosha quiz from Chapter D. Then follow the tips below.

People who have a Vata constitution typically have weak digestion and are least able to tolerate a raw foods diet. Warm, cooked foods are grounding and nourishing. Cooked foods increase Pitta and warm beverages increase Kapha, thereby balancing Vata.

People who have a Pitta constitution typically have strong digestion and are able to tolerate raw foods the best of all the Dosha types. If living in cold, dry climates, however, adding some cooked foods may be beneficial.

People who have a Kapha constitution may have strong or sluggish digestion. If digestion is strong, raw foods will be beneficial. If digestion is weak, cooked foods will be best.

Deepak Chopra suggests the following Ayurvedic tips for better digestion:

- Avoid really cold food and liquids.
- Sip hot water with meals. Drink the majority of your water between meals.
- Include fresh ginger root, lime or lemon juice, and small amounts of fermented foods to increase *Agni* (digestive capacity).
- Include all six tastes—sweet, sour, salty, pungent, bitter, and astringent—in every meal to ensure balance.
- Eat mindfully, taking your time to enjoy your food.
- Eat according to your primary constitution: Vata, Pitta, or Kapha.
- Align yourself with the rhythms of nature. Eat mostly warm, cooked foods when the weather is cool and the qualities of Vata are increased. Salads and other raw foods are best eaten when the weather is hot and at lunchtime—between noon and 2 p.m.—when *Agni* is strongest.
- Incorporate healthy fats and cold-pressed organic oils such as extra-virgin olive oil to balance Vata when consuming salads and dried foods.
- Soak and sprout nuts and seeds to unlock nutrients and increase their digestibility.
- Juice raw vegetables to decrease the element of dryness and reduce the digestive demands on your body. I don't recommend juicing more than one piece of fruit daily as this leads to increased blood sugar levels.
- Include spices that enhance digestion and reduce gas and bloating, such as coriander, cumin, and fennel.
- Practice *Pranayama*. Refer back to the Chapter B video if you need a refresher.

- *Bhastrika* is a simple yogic breathing practice that will help energize you as well as enhance your digestive power. There are several videos online about this.
- Practice yoga poses that massage the abdominal organs, such as gentle twists, reclined knee-to-chest pose, downward dog, and cat-cow pose.

Physical Health

Heat it Up
Hot Towel Scrub

Body scrubbing can be done before or after your bath or shower, or anytime during the day. All you need is a sink with hot water and a medium-sized washcloth (I like to use organic cotton, eucalyptus, or bamboo).

For the maximum effect, scrub your body twice a day: once in the morning and once again in the evening. Scrub for two to twenty minutes, depending on how much time you have. The process of the hot towel scrub has a deeper physical, mental and emotional effect when done at the sink as opposed to in the shower.

Directions:
- Turn on the hot water and fill the sink.
- Hold the towel at both ends and place in the hot water.
- Wring out the towel.
- While the towel is still hot and steamy, begin to scrub the skin gently.
- Do one section of the body at a time: for example, begin with the hands and fingers and work your way up the arms to the shoulders, neck and face, then down to the chest, upper back, abdomen, lower back, buttocks, legs, feet and toes.
- Scrub until the skin becomes slightly pink or until each part becomes warm.
- Reheat the towel often by dipping it in the sink of hot water after scrubbing each section, or as soon as the washcloth starts to cool.

Benefits:
- Reduces muscle tension.
- Reenergizes in the morning and deeply relaxes at night.
- Opens the pores to release stored toxins.
- Softens deposits of hard fat below the skin and prepares them for discharge.

- Allows excess fat, mucus, cellulite and toxins to actively discharge to the surface rather than to accumulate around deeper vital organs.
- Relieves stress through meditative action of rubbing the skin.
- Calms the mind.
- Promotes circulation.
- Activates the lymphatic system, especially when scrubbing underarms and groin.
- Easy massage and deep self-care.
- Can be a relaxing moment in your day, especially if done with candlelight and a drop or two of essential oil, such as lavender.
- Creates a profound and loving relationship with the body, especially parts not often shown care, and especially for a person with body image problems.
- Spreads energy through the chakras.

Hot Water Bottle

Once you use a hot water bottle, you won't believe how you ever got along without it. The hot water bottle is one of the most useful all-purpose health-care products you will ever use. It is designed to apply comfortable, soothing heat therapy easily and conveniently to any part of the body for a variety of ailments.

Fill it with hot water from the sink. The water bottle will stay warm for up to two hours.

Use it to:
- Relax particular muscles or use for the entire body
- Deliver nurturing comfort to enable a deep state of relaxation

Try using the hot water bottle on:
- The feet for warmth
- The back for strain
- The lower abdomen for cramps
- The abdomen for digestion and relaxation of body and mind

Additional uses:
- To combat illness: use as a warm, soothing companion to help you through flu, chills, and aches.

- To ease menstrual cramps: a hot water bottle on the abdomen brings pain relief and soothing comfort.
- As a bed warmer: a warm hot water bottle placed in your bed makes for a cozy sleep, especially on cold winter nights.
- To ease arthritic pain: a natural, moist heat therapy for arthritic pain relief, especially great for hands.
- To calm children: a warm cuddly companion to provide a calm secure feeling when children are ill or upset.
- As a traveling companion: take it with you on trips to comfort you. No electricity needed.
- To calm your pet: placed under a blanket, a warm hot water bottle soothes puppies in new surroundings. It provides warmth and security and calms them down.
- To encourage restful sleep: to help you sleep after a high-stress day, lie down with a hot water bottle on your stomach, close your eyes and breathe deeply, so the bottle rises and falls. Many people carry a lot of tension there and the weighted heat releases it.

Sex

Research indicates that a healthy sex life leads to a longer, healthier, and most would say more enjoyable life. Here are some specific reasons to "heat it up" between the sheets. According to Dr. Joseph Mercola, an osteopathic physician and alternative medicine proponent, here are eleven health benefits of a healthy sex life:

1. **Improved Immunity**

   Having sex one or two times a week has shown to significantly increase levels of immunoglobulin A (IgA). Your IgA immune system is your body's first line of defense. Its job is to fight off invading organisms at their entry points, reducing or even eliminating the need for activation of your body's immune system. This may explain why people who have sex frequently also take fewer sick days.

2. **Heart Health**

   Men who made love regularly—at least twice a week—were 45 percent less likely to develop heart disease than those who did so once a month or less, according to one study. Sexual activity not only provides many of the same benefits to your heart as exercise but also keeps levels of estrogen and testosterone in balance, which is important for heart health.

3. **Lower Blood Pressure**

    Sexual activity, and specifically intercourse, is linked to better stress response and lower blood pressure.

4. **It's a Form of Exercise**

    Sex helps to boost your heart rate, burn calories and strengthen muscles, just like exercise. In fact, research recently revealed that sex burns about four calories a minute for men and three for women, making it a significant form of exercise at times. It can even help you to maintain your flexibility and balance.

5. **Pain Relief**

    Sexual activity releases pain-reducing hormones and has been found to help reduce or block back and leg pain, as well as pain from menstrual cramps, arthritis and headaches. One study even found that sexual activity can lead to partial or complete relief of headaches in some migraine and cluster-headache patients.

6. **May Help Reduce Risk of Prostate Cancer**

    Research has shown that men who ejaculate at least twenty-one times a month—during sex or masturbation—have a lower risk of prostate cancer. This link needs to be explored further, however, as there may have been additional factors involved in the association.

7. **Improve Sleep**

    After sex, the relaxation-inducing hormone prolactin is released, which may help you to nod off more quickly. The "love hormone" oxytocin, released during orgasm, also promotes sleep.

8. **Stress Relief**

    Sex triggers your body to release its natural feel-good chemicals, helping to ease stress and boost pleasure, calm and self-esteem. Research also shows that those who have sexual intercourse responded better when subjected to stressful situations like speaking in public.

9. **Boost Your Libido**

    The more often you have sex, the more likely you are to want to keep doing it. There's a mental connection there but also a physical one, particularly for women. More frequent sex helps to increase vaginal lubrication, blood flow and elasticity, which in turn make sexual activity more enjoyable.

10. **Improved Bladder Control in Women**

    Intercourse helps to strengthen your pelvic floor muscles, which contract during orgasm. This can help women to improve their bladder control and avoid incontinence. You can boost this benefit even more by practicing Kegel exercises during sex. A Kegel squeeze is performed by drawing your lower pelvic muscles up and holding them up high and tight, as if you're trying to stop a flow of urine.

11. **Increase Intimacy and Improve Your Relationship**

    Sex and orgasms result in increased levels of the hormone oxytocin—the "love" hormone—which helps you feel bonded to your partner and better experience empathic connections.

Cognitive Health

Hypnosis

> Check out www.rhondahuff.com for the video lessons,
> "Chapter H Reveal" and "Chapter H Receive"

Sometimes people hear the word "hypnosis" and immediately think it is fake or dangerous. I am not talking about any weird phenomenon or theatrical performances.

Neuroscientists have shown that the conscious mind provides 5 percent or less of our cognitive (conscious) activity during the day. And 5 percent, they say, is for the more aware people. Many people operate at just 1 percent consciousness. American biologist and expert on the power of the subconscious mind Dr. Bruce Lipton says the subconscious mind operates at 40 million bits of data per second, whereas the conscious mind processes at only 40 bits per second. So, the subconscious mind is MUCH more powerful than the conscious mind, and it is the subconscious mind that shapes how we live our life.

As we discussed in Chapter E, TRUE and LASTING change must happen in the subconscious! So, we are taking a stroll all the way back to Chapter A...

I fully love and accept you just as you are right now.

That's right. We have been working on this affirmation since the very beginning. Many of you are still struggling with it. And guess what? I knew that would be the case! So today I am going to walk you through a hypnosis session to get the subconscious to do two things:

1. Reveal the affliction
2. Receive the affirmation

REVEAL will walk you through a session to help you reveal the affliction.

RECEIVE will walk you through a session to help you receive the affirmation.

CHAPTER I PREP

1. Hopefully with all the practice and the Chapter H hypnosis video, you can now look yourself in the eye and say,
   I fully love and accept you just as you are right now.
   Record how you now feel about those words.

   _____

   _____

   _____

2. Begin Chapter I's affirmation (still to be done looking only at your eyes, repeating seven times, morning and night).
   I am making room in my life for what is ideal.

3. Foam roll and do the corrective exercises as a warmup for each workout day this week. And continue to foam roll daily. Remember to record your workouts.

4. Check in with your Circle of Life. This should now be an established habit of working on your action steps. Record your thoughts here:

   _____

   _____

   _____

5. Recognize and handle distress as it pops up this week. Record below.

   _____

   _____

6. How are your eating patterns going? Are you at four hours between meals and a twelve-hour fast between dinner and breakfast? (Remember if you are diabetic, you are to clear all modifications with your doctor.)

7. Remember the Four Agreements

8. Use the FOOD© principle and add prebiotic and probiotic foods into your day.

9. Practice gratitude everyday.

10. Continue to use the hypnosis video to work on revealing afflictions and receiving affirmations. The goal is to be able to self-hypnotize and to use anchors to drive behavior and thought until they become habit. Record your progress here:

_____

_____

_____

CHAPTER I

Emotional Health

Ideal Worksheet

This is a tool for you to create a clear list of what you really want in any and all aspects of your life, be it an apartment, a job, a relationship, a car, or anything else!

Step 1: Pick what it is you want to create and write it on the top. Example: My ideal apartment.

Step 2: List all the things that your ideal must have. THESE ARE YOUR NON-NEGOTIABLES! Be specific. Example: decent-sized bathtub, a big refrigerator, air conditioning, three blocks from the subway, etc.

Step 3: List all the things that your ideal preferably has. THESE ARE YOUR NEGOTIABLES! Example: a dishwasher, a washing machine, an office, wood floors, etc.

Step 4: List all the things that your ideal preferably does not have. THESE ARE YOUR NEGOTIABLES! Example: noisy neighbors, above third floor, etc.

Step 5: List all the things that your ideal must not have. THESE ARE YOUR NON-NEGOTIABLES! Example: mice, roaches, leaks, thin walls, etc.

MY IDEAL_____			
Must have / be	**Preferably** has / is	**Preferably** does not have / is not	**Must** not have / not be

Nutritional Health

Intermittent Fasting

If you have been getting 12 hours between your last meal of the day and your first meal of the day you have been practicing one form of intermittent fasting. An interesting fact is that the only thing that has ever been proven to potentially reduce disease risk and increase life span, is reducing caloric consumption.

Religions worldwide have long maintained the benefits of fasting. Now there is science to back up those claims. Since the early 1900's doctors have been using fasting to deal with obesity, epilepsy, and diabetes and even the more recent research about its benefits date back to the mid 1940's when scientists from the University of Chicago expanded on research that began in the 1930's at Cornell University.

The decades following led to new developments in medicine such as pharmaceuticals and surgery. Now, many medical professionals are beginning to take another look at more holistic ways of dealing with aging and disease. Intermittent fasting is one of those ways.

Here are some health benefits of intermittent fasting (IF):

1. Cellular repair processes improve
2. Fat burning increases
3. Hormone function is enhanced
4. Metabolic rate increases
5. Insulin resistance is reduced
6. Oxidative stress is reduced

7. Inflammation is reduced
8. Blood pressure improves
9. Lipid profiles improve
10. Growth of new nerve cells increases
11. Alzheimer's disease can be delayed or prevented
12. Lifespan increases

Be smart when beginning intermittent fasting that is more than the 12 hour fast you have been doing on this program and consult your physician first. Below are 5 types of popular intermittent fasting methods:

1. The 16/8 Method: fast for 14-16 hours per day and eating during the other 8-10 hours per day. If you are already doing the 12 hour fast and wish to try this, work up to 14-16 hours from your last meal.
2. The 5:2 Method: restrict calories to 500-600 calories for two days out of five per week. For example, you may restrict your calories on Mondays and Thursdays of each week.
3. The Eat-Stop-Eat Method: this is a 24-hour fast that you can do once or twice a week.
4. The Alternate Day Method: staying under 500 calories every other day.
5. Spontaneous Meal Skipping: just listening to your body and choosing to skip a meal here and there from time to time.

Let me reiterate, *consult your physician* before following any of these five intermittent fasting plans. I also do not recommend intermittent fasting to anyone struggling with an eating disorder where food restriction may be a trigger to unhealthy habits. The methods that I feel are the safest are the 12 hour overnight fast, the 16/8 method, the 5:2 method, and the spontaneous meal skipping method.

Physical Health

Interval Training

Check out www.rhondahuff.com for the video lesson, "Chapter I"

Exercise has many benefits such as combatting disease, increasing energy, improving mood, and promoting better sleep, among many others. However, most people would place losing weight as a primary reason to exercise. And though losing weight is a great idea, it is a terrible goal. A goal should be Specific, Measureable, Attainable, Relevant, and Time-specific (SMART). Losing weight is not specific. However, when I push for specifics on this topic I usually get a comeback like "I would like to lose twenty pounds." Ok. So, let's walk through why this isn't a good goal and how interval training can help us reach a great goal.

"I would like to lose twenty pounds"

Problem 1: "I would like" usually indicates an unwillingness to do the work needed to reach the goal. This is a wish, not a goal.

Solution is "I will." This changes the way the brain looks at the statement. It now becomes a priority on a much deeper level.

Problem 2: "Twenty pounds." Twenty pounds of what? If you are only doing cardio and not eating properly that twenty pounds will likely contain a high amount of muscle loss. All of you have seen what this looks like and may have experienced it yourself. It looks like a thinner person who appears flabby and maybe even gaunt, but not healthy and glowing. Even most doctors still use BMI (Body Mass Index) as a gauge of health. The problem with BMI is that two men can have the SAME BMI of 33.9, yet one can be about 5 percent body fat and the other can be about 40 percent body fat. BMI only looks at your height versus your weight. It tells us nothing about your body composition or your health.

Solution is to calculate "___ PERCENT body fat." Depending on the instrument used, this number will vary. The Omron Fat Loss Monitor is what I use. You can find this on the link www.rhondahuff.com. With this monitor, the norms are:

	Age	Low	Ideal	High	Very High
Female	20-39	5-20	21-33	34-38	>38
	40-59	5-22	23-34	35-40	>40
	60-79	5-23	24-36	37-41	>41
Male	20-39	5-7	8-20	21-25	>25
	40-59	5-10	11-21	22-27	>27
	60-79	5-12	13-25	26-30	>30

I recommend getting your body fat percentage to the recommended range. Therefore, if your body fat percentage is 48 and you are a 45-year-old female, I would want your goal to be to get your body fat percentage down to 34, which is the upper limit of the recommended range. (Once you are there then you decide how much more—if any—you need to lose and make a new goal.) To get to recommended range goal, we would set smaller (more attainable to the mind/emotions) goals with timelines. It may look like this:

"Today is April 2, 2016. I will lose 2 percent body fat (46 percent) by April 30, 2016. I will do this by following this plan…"

In order for your goal to be attainable, you must be willing to comply with the plan. Be realistic. Be kind to yourself. We are so brainwashed to think quick results are best. I think permanent results are best.

And that leads me to the wonders of interval training. If you have Kapha or Pitta exercise recommendations then interval training may change your life.

By incorporating intense periods of work with short periods of recovery, interval training will burn body fat and preserve muscle mass. And unlike traditional cardio, doing intervals will keep your body burning fat even after you finish the workout, burning fat calories at a higher rate for up to three days! You may have heard of Excess Post-exercise Oxygen Consumption (EPOC). That's what makes interval training magical. Your body can't deliver enough oxygen to your muscles during periods of hard work and your muscles accumulate a debt of oxygen that must be repaid post-workout in order to get back to normal. This leaves your metabolism revved-up for hours after you finish the workout and assists the body in burning fat for days after. Also, the intensity will stimulate muscle building hormones, allowing you to maintain a better body composition (glowing and healthy instead of flabby and gaunt), and develops the cardiovascular system during the intense work and improves the recovery system during the rest!

So, what if you are a Vata? Can you get this benefit without over-taxing your system and results in an over-accumulation of cortisol, which offsets the benefits? Yes, BUT you should not push yourself to exhaustion or over-stimulation. Relaxing, rhythmic activities balance Vata so keep that in mind as you prepare your interval routine. Incorporate rowing, yoga, dance, weights, tai chi, and outdoor activities on warm days when possible.

You may have noticed that I have not referred to interval training as High Intensity Interval Training (HIIT). This is because I am not a fan of many of the HIIT models out there. I prefer you look at your own individual body and decide how intense your work should be and how long your recovery should be. Keep in mind that we usually won't push ourselves beyond our perceived comfort zones and our perceived comfort zones are typically out of the range of effective exercise. Hiring a qualified trainer to help you discern what your appropriate levels are is smart. I won't get on my soapbox about what qualified means but I do suggest you do some research before hiring one. If you hire a trainer because they have "worked out their whole lives" or just because they have a great body, you may want to reconsider. RESEARCH!

Guidelines for Interval Training:
Intensity: 80 to 95 percent of your estimated Maximum Heart Rate (MHR).

To keep things simple, we will use the standard MHR formula of 220 minus your age. There are many formulas out there and a clinical determination is always best. However, the American College of Sports Medicine is still the gold standard for exercise guidelines and they still use this formula.

220 minus your age = MHR
Your MHR is _____ This is the number you do not want to go above.

Now determine the intensity. These two numbers will be your range for the **intense portion** of interval training.

Your MHR * .80 =
Your MHR * .95 =

And determine the recovery. These two numbers will be your range for the **recovery portion** of interval training.

Your MHR * .40 =
Your MHR * .50 =

Monitor your heart rate for both portions. Your recovery time continues until your heart rate has dropped between those two numbers. *RECOVERY IS AS IMPORTANT AS WORK!* There are hundreds of interval programs online. Some do a 1:1 work/recovery ratio, some do a 1:3, etc. Just do what you enjoy and what you can do with proper form!

The workout continues for fifteen to sixty minutes. This is another reason I don't use the term "HIIT" as most HIIT proponents state that if you can sustain interval training for more than ten to twenty minutes, you aren't really doing HIIT and aren't working hard enough. While that is a valid argument, safety comes first. Find your own comfort zone and improve from there.

Keep track of how the recovery times shorten! This is where you will know you are making progress!

And remember that practice makes PERMANENT. Only PERFECT practice makes perfect. Proper form and exercise execution MUST take priority over any other factor.

So, let's give this a try…

Your favorite lower body exercise:

_____

_____

_____

Your favorite upper body exercise:

_____

_____

_____

Your favorite core (think entire core, not just abs) exercise:

_____

_____

_____

Your favorite metabolic exercise (something that gets your heart rate up like jumping rope or jogging or lateral shuffles):

_____

_____

_____

Now create an interval routine with it!

I like to work in threes so I would do Lower Body, Upper Body, and either Core or Metabolic. I then repeat it two more times so that I have completed a circuit of three exercises three times.

Now do it again:

Lower Body:

_____

_____

_____

Upper Body:

_____

_____

_____

Core:

_____

_____

_____

Metabolic:

_____

_____

_____

And once more!

Lower Body:

_____

_____

_____

Upper Body:

_____

_____

_____

Core:

_____

_____

_____

Metabolic:

_____

_____

_____

Now you have a full one-hour format if you so choose. Here is what it looks like:

1. Foam Roll
2. Warm-up (can be correctives if you haven't mastered them)
3. Circuit 1
4. Circuit 2
5. Circuit 3
6. Stretch and/or Foam Roll again

Here is how to determine estimated repetitions (reps):

- For strength keep the reps at ten or below
- For hypertrophy (muscle mass) keep the reps between ten and fifteen
- For weight loss keep the reps between fifteen and twenty

NOTE: I train everyone for strength first. This way I can perfect form without them getting fatigued and losing proper form. I suggest you do the same for the first four to six weeks.

Now here is where your interval knowledge comes in.

CIRCUIT 1

Do the first exercise and record your pulse:

_____

Do the second exercise and record your pulse:

_____

Do the third exercise and record your pulse:

_____

Now rest until your pulse is in the recovery range.

CIRCUIT 2

Do the first exercise and record your pulse:

_____

Do the second exercise and record your pulse:

_____

Do the third exercise and record your pulse:

_____

Now rest until your pulse is in the recovery range.

CIRCUIT 3

Do the first exercise and record your pulse:

_____

Do the second exercise and record your pulse:

_____

Do the third exercise and record your pulse:

_____

Now rest until your pulse is in the recovery range.

Cognitive Health

Intuition

Scientific American defines intuition as "the name we give to the uncanny ability to quickly and effortlessly know the answer, unconsciously, either without or well before knowing why. The conscious explanation comes later, if at all, and involves a much more deliberate process." Physicists and chemists are said to rely on intuition in formulating theories and formulas. It is rumored that Albert Einstein (known as one of the greatest intuitives of his time) had this saying in his office, "Not everything that can be counted counts, and not everything that counts can be counted."

By all practical definitions, I am a scientist. I need proof. I need whys. I need constants. I research the research and I research the researchers. If the researchers have a vested interest in the outcome—as they often do—I will not put much clout into the results that are claimed. Furthermore, I will listen to anyone's opinion, but my comeback usually is, "OK. Prove it to me." If you can prove it, I will instantly change my stance. I have done it many times. If you can't prove it, then it is like you are talking to a brick wall because I will not budge.

And just as I love the quote that may or may not have actually been on Einstein's office wall, his colleague, physicist Richard Feynman said, "The first principle is that you must not fool yourself, and you are the easiest person to fool."

For example, you suddenly think of a friend and give her a call only to discover she was in a car accident at the very moment she had come to mind. Or, you go to a different grocery store and later learn there was a shooting at your regular grocery store at the time you would have been there. Or, perhaps, you are walking through the park and all of a sudden, the hair seems to stand up on the back of your neck. You abort your plans and leave the park just before a rash of robberies take place there. Are these examples of intuition, fortunate coincidences, God's protection, or a combination of these things?

And then we have these: You feel unusually lucky, so you spend $20 on Power Ball tickets and do not get a single number. You thought you were getting fired and prepared your battle speech but instead were given an unexpected promotion. Your son was late for curfew and didn't answer your calls and you just knew he was in serious trouble, but he was fine and just being rebellious. Are these examples of intuition gone wrong or simply life in motion?

And my favorite personal example: I know people who just simply "know" where they are in the world. I, on the other hand, stay lost most of the time. This is so predictable for me that if my intuition says to go right, I most certainly should go left. So, what do I make of my own intuition being that it has led me astray so many times?

Therefore, intuition is a subject that tends to perplex me. Can it be proven? Is the research consistent? Where do the fields of psychology and science merge on the subject, if they do at all? Turns out that scientists who study intuition say it's a very real ability that can be identified in lab experiments and visualized on brain scans.

If you Google intuition you will find hundreds of examples and research articles supporting intuition as reliable AND supporting intuition as unreliable. So how do we decipher all the information and make use of knowledge? Perhaps *Psychology Today* says it best in the article titled "The Powers and Perils of Intuition."

"Instinct has the power to hush reason. But when is it safe to go with your gut? Researchers may remain uncertain about the reliability of intuition, but it is a difficult force to deny."

The article goes on to explore "dual processing," which is what we engage when we do the hypnosis sections of the program. Our thoughts, memories and attitudes operate on two levels: the conscious/deliberate and the unconscious/subconscious/automatic. We most definitely know more than we think we do.

Psychologists John Bargh, Ph.D., of New York University and Tanya Chartrand, Ph.D., of Ohio State University say, "Our consciousness is biased to think that its own intentions and deliberate choices rule our lives. But consciousness overrates its own control." In his research, Bargh discovered that when his students were shown flashes of photos for only two-tenths of a second, an evaluation as to whether the image was good or bad happened within a quarter of a second, which is long before rational thought kicks in.

"Indeed, thanks to emotional pathways that run from the eye to the brain's emotional control centers—bypassing the cortex—we often react emotionally before we've even had time to interpret consciously. Below the radar of awareness, we can process threatening information in milliseconds. Then, after the cortex has had time to interpret the threat, the thinking brain asserts itself. In the forest, we physically jump at the sound of rustling leaves, leaving the cortex to decide later whether the sound came from a predator or the wind."

The perils of intuition are also very real. We often over predict how yummy food will be tomorrow if we are shopping while hungry today. We also think the devastation from things such as break-ups or arguments will last longer than they really do.

This occurs because people neglect the speed and power of their "psychological immune system," which includes strategies for rationalizing, discounting, forgiving, and limiting trauma. Being ignorant of this emotional recovery system, we accommodate illnesses, disabilities, romantic breakups, and defeats more readily than we intuitively expect.

My take on all this? It's about balance. Should we trust our intuition more? Probably. Should we then use rational thought to support or reject that intuition? Probably. I can say that I wish I had used my intuition more in the past. I over-analyze a lot. And that can be exhausting and often leads to indecision, which in and of itself is a decision, a decision of inaction.

When you improve your intuition, you will become more observant of your own mind and of your surroundings. This can lead to fewer mistakes, an improved ability to make decisions throughout the day, and increased creativity and problem-solving abilities.

Here are a few ways to improve your ability to use the power of your intuition:

- **Learn to be still.** Only in stillness can we weed through the chatter and chaos of life.
- **Write down your thoughts.** Journaling allows you to center in on what is bothering you, what is important to you, and what may be preventing progress in other areas of your life.
- **Make health a priority.** When you are exhausted and unhealthy the intuition cannot work optimally.
- **Pray or meditate.** Prayer and meditation is proven to alleviate stress and help the mind focus on positive change and improved mood.
- **Follow the Four Agreements,** especially "Don't make assumptions." Intuition is not synonymous with assumption. We make assumptions when we try to force an answer to something we are unsure about. Assumptions are often unfair assessments of people or situations. Intuition is based on the desire for truth and has no room for assumptive thinking.

What will you commit to this week to improve your intuition? Comment and track below:

_____

_____

_____

CHAPTER J PREP

1. Begin Chapter J's affirmation (still to be done looking only at your eyes, repeating seven times, morning and night).
   I am healthy in mind and body.
2. Foam roll and do the corrective exercises as a warmup for each workout day this week. And continue to foam roll daily. Remember to record your workouts.
3. Recognize and handle distress as it pops up this week. Record below.

_____

4. How are your eating patterns going? Are you at four hours between meals and a twelve-hour fast between dinner and breakfast? (Remember if you are diabetic, you are to clear all modifications with your doctor.)
5. Remember the Four Agreements
6. Use the FOOD© principle and add prebiotic and probiotic foods into your day.
7. Practice gratitude everyday.
8. Continue to use the hypnosis video to work on revealing afflictions and receiving affirmations. The goal is to be able to self-hypnotize and to use

anchors to drive behavior and thought until they become habit. Record your progress here:

_____

_____

_____

9. Have you used your Ideal Worksheet to help with decision-making yet? If so, how did that go?

_____

_____

_____

10. Did you try a new intermittent fasting method? If so, how did it go?

_____

_____

_____

CHAPTER J

Emotional Health

Journaling

We have touched on journaling and the importance of getting your thoughts on paper. But why is it so important for emotional health? Oscar Wilde, 19th-century playwright, said: "I never travel without my diary. One should always have something sensational to read on the train." Your life is sensational. Your experiences are sensational. YOU are sensational. Journaling allows us not only to work through difficult thoughts and feelings but also allows us to record our daily adventures, our struggles, successes, times of sorrow and happiness. If you have ever looked back over past journals it is likely that you have had these types of reactions: "Oh, my gosh! I forgot about that! That was so much fun!" "Wow, I didn't realize that I have been unhappy about this for so long." "Yikes, I see so much of what my child is going through right now in this journal! I forgot how difficult this time of life can be."

Here is a bit of research about journaling:

- Regular journaling strengthens immune cells, called T-lymphocytes. (University of Texas at Austin, James Pennebaker)
- Journaling decreases the symptoms of asthma and rheumatoid arthritis. ((University of Texas at Austin, James Pennebaker)

- The act of writing uses your left brain, which is analytical and rational. While your left brain is occupied with writing, your right brain is free to create, intuit and feel. Writing opens the creative pathway and removes mental blocks we experience when only "thinking through things." "Writing through things" leads to more solutions and happier outcomes by helping clarify and organize thoughts and creative solutions.
- Journaling allows you to get to know yourself better.
- Journaling reduces stress.
- Journaling allows you to say things that you would like to say to others but know you shouldn't. Writing the hateful and destructive words down allows you to process the emotions BEFORE actually dealing with the person who has upset you. The book "Lincoln on Leadership" states that Lincoln wrote many letters and never sent them for this very reason.

There are many types of journals and ways to journal. Decide what appeals to you and give it a try. Also, you don't have to journal every day so don't fall into the trap of perfectionism. Sometimes we feel like if we can't do something perfectly then we should just quit altogether. This is destructive. Remember this journey is a process. Trust the process.

Early Morning Pages. This type of journaling is done at that small moment when you first wake up in the morning. This moment is when most people fall back to sleep for a few more precious minutes. But this moment is a powerful moment to journal. If you can pull yourself out of bed at that moment and journal, you may discover some interesting things. I had a lady who couldn't figure out why she was so unhappy and by doing early morning pages realized it was her job. She found a new job and found the happiness that had eluded her for so many years. Here is what you do:

- Write down any portion of dreams that you remember.
- Write down any words or phrases that are in your mind upon awakening.

Initially it may appear to be a jumbled mess. With time, patterns will emerge. It's a fascinating tool and the people I know who have used it have had tremendous success with it. The biggest hurdle is simply making yourself choose journaling over a few more minutes of sleep.

Personal Development Journal. This type of journal is a way to track your growth as a person. The Circle of Life is a great tool to use with this journal as it shows you areas of your life that you already know you want to improve. And over time you will be able to see how much you have grown and changed. I would encourage you to be specific about the topics in this journal. You may want to title your journal entries with specific topics such as Career, Spirituality, Relationships, Physical Activity, Education, etc.

Project Journal. If you have a hard time completing projects, this can be an effective tool to keep you on track and moving forward.

Gratitude Journal. We practiced this in Chapter G. It is a powerful tool in keeping us focused on our blessings instead of our burdens.

Your Choice. This, ultimately, is your journey so make up your own journal. There are no rules to follow. Just write.

Nutritional Health

Juicing

Juicing is a trendy topic at the moment. Everywhere you look people are sipping on smoothies and juices. There seems to be a great divide between the people who love juicing and the people who hate it. I will provide some clarity on both sides. But first, I want to be very specific on what type of juicing I am discussing—**VEGETABLE** juicing.

Most people juice their fruits and maybe throw in a small dose of green. This is NOT healthy! Juicing fruits concentrates the sugars way too much. If you want fruit, EAT it in moderation but don't drink it. The only fruit you should add to your juice is lemon, lime, or cranberries, which have negligible fructose.

Blending or Juicing? Is there a difference?

Yes. Blenders—and also centrifugal juicers—heat up the vegetables, which destroy the very enzymes and nutrients we want to provide the body. This negates the whole purpose of juicing. Get a single-gear or twin-gear juicer if you truly want to juice for health. If you don't want to juice for health, just eat your food instead and forget about juices and smoothies.

But blenders preserve the fiber, right?

Yes, they do. But once again, the purpose of juicing is to nourish the body in the most effective way. If you are going for micronutrients, juicing will allow you to get more vegetables into the body. The fiber content of blending won't allow you to get enough because it will fill you up too quickly. Also, it's the pulp that makes vegetable smoothies taste gross. Plus, the heat will destroy many of the nutrients anyway. Save and store the fiber though. You can add it to recipes to increase the nutrient and fiber content of other foods such as muffins.

Who should juice?

Most people should NOT juice his or her meals. Vegetable juice is not a complete meal as it has very little protein and virtually no fat. And even though you can add protein and Medium Chain Triglycerides (MCT oil) to help with this, your juice should be used in addition to your regular meals not in place of it. And even though I know people who juice daily, you need to decide what works best for you.

People with irritable bowel syndrome, Crohn's disease, and other kinds of gastrointestinal problems can usually handle vegetable juice because it doesn't need to be digested, the fiber has been extracted, and the nutrients are quickly delivered to the body.

And just a reminder that green vegetables are high in vitamin K so if you are on an anticoagulant please consult your doctor before juicing to determine how much you can safely consume.

IMPORTANT: Only juice ORGANIC vegetables! Otherwise you will be ingesting a pesticide cocktail! Gross!

If you are new to juicing, the easiest ones are usually

- Celery
- Fennel
- Cucumbers

The next level would be

- Red or green leaf lettuce
- Romaine lettuce
- Endive
- Escarole
- Spinach
- Cabbage (great for ulcer repair)

Then add some herbs, staring with

- Cilantro
- Parsley

And finally, once you have mastered the above, add the more bitter veggies

- Kale
- Collards (should still be attached to the stalk for best nutrient value)
- Dandelion greens
- Mustard greens
- And if you want a little kick, add some heart-healthy fresh ginger

Physical Health

Joints

Check out www.rhondahuff.com for the video lesson, "Chapter J"

Now that you have had time to reap the many benefits of Self Myofascial Release and Corrective Exercise, it is time to check in with your joints.

We will start from the ground up.

Stability: the ability to maintain or control joint movement or position

Mobility: the range of uninhibited movement around a joint

Joint / Purpose	Is this joint fulfilling its purpose without complaint (pain)?	If no, explain
Foot / Stability		
Ankle / Mobility		
Knee / Stability		
Hip / Mobility		

Lumbar Spine (low back) / Stability		
Thoracic Spine (between shoulder blades) / Mobility		
Scapulae (shoulder blades) / Stability		
Glenohumeral Joint (shoulders) / Mobility		
Lower Cervical Spine / Stability		
Upper Cervical Spine / Mobility		

If you are still having pain or are not getting the proper stability or mobility at a specific joint, it is important to determine why. Have you done the foam rolling and correctives as instructed? If not, try to make a plan to be compliant in this area. If yes, consider the following questions. Was there a previous injury? Have you had surgery that wasn't rehabilitated properly? Do you have connective tissue that is torn? Is there scar tissue that prevents proper movement? Get curious. Call a doctor. Don't settle for less than optimal health. You must be your own advocate.

Cognitive Health

Juggling
Juggling? Really? Yes! Believe it or not, juggling is a great brain exercise. And it is also a fun stress-reliever if you can drop the expectations and just laugh your way through it!

Why is juggling—or attempting to juggle—so good for your brain?

- Improves hand-eye coordination
- Improves reflexes
- Improves peripheral vision
- Sharpens concentration
- Increases neuronal activity in the brain
- Increases gray matter in two areas of the brain involved in visual and motor activity, the mid-temporal area and the posterior intraparietal sulcus (this study was done after three months of juggling, however after three more

months of not juggling, the increase in size decreased, supporting the theory that if you don't use it you lose it)

Lifehack.org gives the following suggestions for learning to juggle.

- Get the basic "feel" of the process by throwing a ball in an arc from one hand to the other; it should rise up to eye height at the peak of its arc.
- A great method to perfect juggling is "scooping", a technique that smooths out your movements. Scoop your hands when throwing back and forth as it greatly helps with overall fluidity.
- Now, with one juggling ball in each hand, throw one in an arc towards your other hand. When it is at the top of its arc lower your other arm to launch the other ball towards your free hand. As each follows its arc catch them in your hands. Practice this to increase your understanding of the motions involved.
- Now try for the three-ball cascade; hold two juggling balls in your right hand, and one in your left. As practiced in point three, throw one ball in a sweeping arc from your right hand. When it has reached the peak of its arc, send the ball in your left hand to your right.
- Catch the first ball in your left hand whilst the second is arching upwards towards your right, now launch the third ball in your right hand towards the left and prepare to catch the second.

CHAPTER K PREP

1. Begin Chapter K's affirmation (still to be done looking only at your eyes, repeating seven times, morning and night).
    I am learning to be kind to others and myself.
2. By now, cravings should be under control most of the time (random cravings will pop up occasionally but should be the exception and not the norm). If cravings are still a constant problem, use the Journaling exercise from Chapter J to uncover what may be emotionally driving the cravings.
3. Foam roll daily and before workouts. Do only the corrective exercises that are still difficult for you.
4. Recognize and handle distress as it pops up this week. Record below.

    _____

    _____

    _____

5. Continue to use the hypnosis video to work on revealing afflictions and receiving affirmations. The goal is to be able to self-hypnotize and to use anchors to drive behavior and thought until they become habit. Record your progress here:

    _____

    _____

    _____

6. Continue using the journal format that is best for you. What have you noticed so far? Has anything changed for you?

    _____

    _____

    _____

7. Did you try a vegetable juice? What did you think?

    _____

    _____

    _____

8. Have you gotten the hang of juggling? If not, keep at it!

CHAPTER K

Emotional Health

Kindness

How often do you go out of your way to be kind to someone? Granted, it is important to be kind as we go about our daily activities and it makes us feel good to hold a door or to smile at someone and that kindness is returned to us with a "thank you" or a smile back. But how often do you actually sacrifice something to be kind to someone? This may be a sacrifice of time, energy, or money. We only have so much of those things available to us in a day, right?

Research shows that when we act kindly to others we reap tremendous health benefits.

- Anxiety and depression are decreased
- Oxytocin is released, which reduces blood pressure due to dilation of blood vessels
- Life satisfaction and overall happiness is increased
- Self-obsession and selfishness are decreased
- Bonding with other people, even strangers, is improved
- And...it is contagious and often causes a positive chain of reactions!

This week commit to one sacrificial act of kindness each day and record below:

Day	Act	How it made me feel
1		
2		
3		
4		
5		
6		
7		

Nutritional Health

Kitchen Cleanup

Cleaning the kitchen can sometimes feel overwhelming but is so satisfying when complete. This week, take a few minutes every day or plan a few hours on one day to clean your kitchen. Here are some basic tips.

Refrigerator/Freezer
- Pull everything out and toss spoiled food and expired condiments into the trash or compost.
- Take removable shelves out and clean with a mix of 1:1 vinegar and water.
- Wipe down inside with your vinegar/water solution.
- Use toothbrush and vinegar/water solution to scrub around the door and crevices of the rubber seal.
- Put good food back.
- Move fridge away from the wall and unplug it.
- Remove the panel that covers the refrigerator coils, and use your vacuum's arm attachment to clean off the dust. Replace the panel and plug in the fridge.
- Clean floor, walls, and sides of fridge before pushing fridge back into place.
- Clean outside of fridge.

Food Cabinets/Pantry
- Pull everything out and toss the following:
- Anything with expired dates
- Anything with anti-nutrients (refer to Chapter F)

- Use your vinegar/water solution to wipe down the shelves and the insides and outsides of cabinet doors.
- Put back remaining food.

Other Cabinets: If doing this daily, choose one or two cabinets or drawers per day until all is done
- Pull everything out.
- Inspect each item and rewash anything that needs it.
- Toss any broken or unused items.
- Wash all caddies, lazy Susans, and other interior organizers.
- Use your vinegar/water solution to wipe down the insides and outsides of cabinets and drawers.
- Replace liners if needed.
- Put back cleaned items.

Dishwasher
- Empty any dishes and remove the racks. Give them a scrub with a toothbrush dipped in your vinegar/water solution. Set aside to dry.
- Use toothbrush and vinegar/water solution to scrub around the door and crevices of the rubber seal.
- Use a clean rag dipped in your vinegar/water solution and wipe down the entire inside of the dishwasher, including the top.
- Scrub the area around the drain, removing any debris or food that's collected down there.
- Replace the racks.
- Clean the outside surface of the dishwasher.
- **Microwave**
- Remove and wash plates and racks.
- Use a clean rag dipped in your vinegar/water solution and wipe down the entire inside of the microwave, including the top.
- Replace the plates and racks.
- Clean the outside surface of the microwave.

Stove/Oven (this takes twelve hours or overnight so plan accordingly)
- Remove and clean all racks, burners, and drip pans.

- Clean underneath the stovetop and the stovetop. Replace drip pans and burners.
- Forgo the toxic fumes and high heat of self-cleaning ovens and unsafe products. Use this idea instead.
  - **What You Need**
    Baking soda
    Damp dishcloth
    Plastic or silicone spatula
    Rubber gloves
    Spray bottle
    Water
    White vinegar
  - **Instructions**
    ◊ **Remove the oven racks:** Remove your oven racks, pizza stone, oven thermometer, and anything else you have inside the oven. Clean them separately.
    ◊ **Make a baking soda paste:** In a small bowl, mix a half cup of baking soda with a few tablespoons of water. Adjust the ratio of both as needed until you have a spreadable paste. For me this took about three tablespoons of water to get the desired spreadable consistency.
    ◊ **Coat your oven:** Spread the paste all over the interior surfaces of your oven, steering clear of the heating elements. I used gloves for this portion, as my oven was pretty grimy. It helped me really get in there and coat the dirtiest nooks and crannies without having to worry about all that grime under my nails. The baking soda will turn a brownish color as you rub it in; it also might be chunkier in some places than others. That is fine. Just try to coat the whole oven to the best of your abilities, paying attention to any particularly greasy areas.
    ◊ **Let it sit overnight:** Allow the baking soda mixture to rest for at least twelve hours, or overnight.
    ◊ **Clean your oven racks:** Meanwhile, clean your oven racks.
    ◊ **Wipe out the oven:** After twelve hours or overnight, take a damp dish cloth and wipe out as much of the dried baking soda paste as you can. Use a plastic or silicone spatula to help scrape off the paste

as needed. I found that the damp cloth was enough for me, but a spatula might come in handy in those hard-to- reach places.

◊ **Spray a little vinegar:** Put a little vinegar in a spray bottle and spritz everywhere you still see baking soda residue in your oven. The vinegar will react with the baking soda and gently foam.

◊ **Do a final wipe down:** Take your damp cloth and wipe out the remaining foamy vinegar-baking-soda mixture. Repeat until all the baking soda residue is gone. Add more water or vinegar to your cloth as needed while wiping to really get the oven clean and shiny.

◊ **Replace your oven racks:** Replace the oven racks and anything else you keep in your oven.

• Clean outside surface of stove.

Sink/Garbage Disposal

• Thoroughly rinse out your sink. If you have a stainless sink, salt and acid in food can potentially damage the finish, so it's important to rinse food and liquids to prevent pitting.

• Sprinkle baking soda onto the surface. Working it into a paste, rinse thoroughly.

• Line the sink with paper towels soaked in white vinegar. Allow it to sit for 20 minutes and then dispose of the paper towels.

• Rinse the sink with warm soapy water.

• For the faucets and handles, wipe with a mild soapy solution. The toothbrush can be used to get in the hard-to-reach areas. If spots remain, a cloth soaked in white vinegar can be used. Once you're finished cleaning, thoroughly rinse once more time and dry with a soft rag. Your sink should now be fresh and clean!

• Sprinkle a half cup of baking soda down the disposal then add one cup of white vinegar. The mixture will fizz and make a bit of noise, allow this to work for a few minutes while you boil a kettle of hot water. Pour boiling water down the drain.

• Fill the drain with two cups of ice. Pour a cup of salt (rock salt is great if you have it, I improvised with coarse sea salt) over the ice cubes. Run the cold water and turn on the garbage disposal until the ice is gone. The ice/salt mixture will help loosen the grime and debris from the grinding elements.

- Cut a lemon or lime in half. With the water on and garbage disposal running, add the fruit halves, one at a time, to the disposal. The fruit will help clean and deodorize your drain.

Countertops/Tables/Light Fixtures/Walls/Floors
- Wipe down countertops, tables, light fixtures, and walls.
- Clean all items on counters and find new homes for items that aren't needed on the countertop.
- Place remaining items back on countertops.
- Sweep floors.
- Mop with the recommended cleaner for your floor. Choose the healthiest version possible.

Stand back and enjoy your masterpiece! Take a deep breath.

Physical Health

Kyphosis

Check out www.rhondahuff.com for the video lesson, "Chapter K"

There are many types of kyphosis. Here is a brief summary:

Osteoporosis-related kyphosis is kyphosis caused from vertebral fracture due to osteoporosis. This can occur in both men and women, but is more common in females. If the vertebrae fractures, it typically occurs in a wedge shape causing the front of the bone to collapse. That segment of the spine then tips forward, resulting in an excessive kyphotic curve and forward stooped posture.

Congenital kyphosis presents itself in infancy or early childhood, due to a malformation of the spinal column in the womb. Usually requires surgery.

Degenerative kyphosis develops due to wear and tear on the spine over time. The underlying cause of the kyphosis typically is spinal arthritis with degeneration of the discs.

Neuromuscular kyophosis occurs due to certain neuromuscular disorders, such as cerebral palsy, spina bifida, or muscular dystrophy.

Nutritional kyphosis is caused by certain vitamin deficiencies during childhood, such as a vitamin D deficiency.

Postural kyphosis is primarily caused by poor posture and slouching. It occurs in people of all ages.

Scheuermann's Disease is due to abnormal growth of the spine and discs. It may become clinically evident in adolescents or adults and is more common in males. Patients typically also have a mild scoliosis. Curves greater than seventy degrees may require surgery.

Traumatic kyphosis results from a misaligned healing of a spinal fracture or injury to the supporting ligaments of the spine.

Iatrogenic kyphosis. "Iatrogenic" means "as a result of medical intervention," and refers to kyphosis developing as a complication of surgical treatment of the spine.

Proper nutrition and exercise can greatly improve or even correct most cases of kyphosis. If you have kyphosis, work on your posture. It will help you move better, breathe better, and feel better!

Cognitive Health

Kryptonite for the Brain

The only research really proving the prevention of conditions like Alzheimer's disease shows that exercise and nutrition is key. For years we thought that puzzles and brain exercises would prevent the degeneration of brain cells but that largely has been discounted in recent years. So, the short answer for keeping your brain healthy is to eat properly and move your body.

There are, however, many things that negatively affect the brain, killing the very brain cells we so desperately want to protect. This is not an exhaustive list.

Remember that balance is important. We can't always have perfect sleep, perfect air quality, and perfect nutrition. However, if you constantly bombard your body with the following, you need to realize that your brain is another organ that is being negatively affected.

- Air pollution
- Artificial sweeteners
- Carbon dioxide poisoning (covering your head while you sleep)
- Cholesterol that is too high or too low
- Chronic stress

- Cigarettes (causes neural inflammation)
- Concussions
- Dehydration or overhydration (think half your body weight in ounces as a good guide)
- Diets too low in good fats
- Heavy metals
- High blood sugar
- Lack of mental stimulation (learn something new, read, practice memorization)
- Lyme disease
- Malnutrition (improper nutrition/too much junk food)
- Negative thought patterns ("stinking thinking")
- No social life
- Not enough exercise
- Overeating
- PTSD
- Sleep deprivation
- Steroids
- Too much alcohol (alcoholics have decreased brain volume)
- Too much gluten or lectins
- Toxic household cleaners

CHAPTER L PREP

1. Begin Chapter L's affirmation (still to be done looking only at your eyes, repeating seven times, morning and night).
   I am learning to speak the love languages of others.
2. Foam roll daily and before workouts. Do only the corrective exercises that are still difficult for you. After foam rolling, use a dynamic warmup before beginning your workout.
3. Recognize and handle distress as it pops up this week. Record below.

   _____

   _____

   _____

4. Continue to use the hypnosis video to work on revealing afflictions and receiving affirmations. The goal is to be able to self-hypnotize and to use anchors to drive behavior and thought until they become habit. Record your progress here:

   _____

   _____

   _____

5. Continue using the journal format that is best for you. What have you noticed so far? Has anything changed for you?

   _____

   _____

6. Did you try a vegetable juice? What did you think?
7. Have you gotten the hang of juggling? If not, keep at it!
8. Is your kitchen clean and organized? Doesn't it feel great?
9. Do you feel kinder and maybe a bit happier after last week? Continue to bless others anytime you can!

CHAPTER L

Emotional Health

Love Languages

One of the most powerful tools I have learned is the concept of Love Languages. The five Love Languages was created by Gary Chapman and explains that with relationships, you can be showing someone love and they may not recognize it for the simple fact that you are speaking the wrong language. Have you ever stopped to think that what makes you feel loved could be completely different from what makes your spouse or anyone else in your life feel loved?

Here is a short description of the five Love Languages:

Acts of Service: To this person, actions speak louder than words. When someone does something for them out of devotion and not duty, it means the world.

Gifts: To this person, a well-thought-out gift shows that someone cares. It is the effort and love behind the gift that is important, not the gift itself.

Physical Touch: To this person, nothing speaks more deeply than appropriate touch. High fives, pats on the back, and hugs go a long way.

Quality Time: To this person, having someone's undivided attention or doing an activity together shows love.

Words of Affirmation: To this person, having someone edify and affirm who they are and/or what they do equals love. Insults cut deeply and are not quickly forgotten.

So, what could this look like? Let's say that Susie is a wonderful servant. She gives of her time and resources regularly. If someone needs a meal cooked, a house cleaned, or an errand run, Susie is your gal! But one day Susie confides in you that she just doesn't feel loved at home. You are shocked! Susie's family is one of the most loving and stable families you know. How could this be true? Susie goes on to explain that no one in her house ever does anything. She cooks. She cleans. She takes out the trash. In order for anyone else to help her, she has to ask. She feels like she does all these things to make her family feel loved and yet gets no reciprocation.

Susie's love language is most likely Acts of Service. Since it is what makes her feel loved, she naturally speaks that language to show others love. But what happens if her husband's love language is Words of Affirmation? How would he naturally show love to Susie? Most likely he (let's call him Sam) would praise her and thank her and express what a great job SHE does with all those things she does for her family. But Susie doesn't feel loved this way. Susie wants Sam to stop praising and start DOING.

But wait...there's more! When Sam DOES do something, usually after being asked by Susie, he needs to be affirmed! He needs to be told what a wonderful job he did and how much she appreciates him and how valuable his help is around the house. It is only then that both Susie and Sam feel loved.

This week, take some time to figure out the love language of everyone who lives in your house. Find the quiz here: *http://www.5lovelanguages.com*

Family Member	Primary Love Language	Secondary Love Language

Nutritional Health

Leaky Gut Syndrome

Dr. Andrew Weil, a Harvard-trained physician and author who has popularized alternative and integrative medicine, states. "Leaky gut syndrome is not generally recognized by conventional physicians, but evidence is accumulating that it is a real condition that affects the lining of the intestines. The theory is that leaky gut syndrome—also called increased intestinal permeability—is the result of damage to the intestinal lining, making it less able to protect the internal environment as well as to filter needed nutrients and other biological substances. As a consequence, some bacteria and their toxins, incompletely digested proteins and fats, and waste not normally absorbed may 'leak' out of the intestines into the blood stream. This triggers an autoimmune reaction, which can lead to gastrointestinal problems such as abdominal bloating, excessive gas and cramps, fatigue, food sensitivities, joint pain, skin rashes, and autoimmunity. The cause of this syndrome may be chronic inflammation, food sensitivity, damage from taking large amounts of nonsteroidal anti-inflammatory drugs (NSAIDS), cytotoxic drugs and radiation or certain antibiotics, excessive alcohol consumption, or compromised immunity."

Here are common symptoms of leaky gut:

Anxiety, arthritis, asthma, auto-immune diseases, bloating, celiac disease, chronic halitosis, Crohn's disease, constipation, diarrhea, depression, eczema, food allergies, gas, Hashimoto's thyroiditis, infertility, insomnia, migraines, psoriasis, rashes, Type 1 or Type 2 diabetes

If you suspect that you may have a leaky gut, there are a few things you can try to get it under control.

Try the GAPS diet, the Specific Carbohydrate Diet (SCD), or the Body Ecology Diet (BED)—what these diets have in common is the **removal** of problematic foods such as gluten, hard-to-digest grains, legumes, sugars, and starches and **adds in** healing foods such as bone-broths, pasture-raised/grass fed meats, organically grown vegetables, healing fats, and fermented foods.

If you want to try it on your own, simply cut out the problematic foods listed above and add in the healthy foods listed below. For most people symptoms will clear in three to six months.

Bone-broth (stock) made from chicken, beef, or other meat bones
Bone broth is full of soothing gelatin and is full of easily digested minerals.

Pasture-raised / grass-fed meats / grass-finished meats
Can be very healing when the cuts involve bone and fat and are slow-cooked or braised.
Naturally cultured or fermented foods

Easily absorbed and full of micro- and macro-nutrients. Examples are vegetables (sauerkraut, kimchi), fruits (chutneys, preserved fruits), beverages (water kefir, kombucha, beet kvass), grains (sourdough bread), dairy (dairy kefir, yogurt, crème fraiche, sour cream), condiments (homemade ketchup, fish sauce, tamari, fermented salsa). There are many tutorials available online teaching how to properly ferment your own foods.

Physical Health

Laughter

Check out www.rhondahuff.com for the video lesson, "Chapter L"

A cheerful disposition is good for your health;
gloom and doom leave you bone-tired.
—Proverbs 17:22 The Message (MSG)

Laughter is good for your mental, social, and physical health. It is, however, fundamentally a physical action. "Laughter involves the repeated, forceful exhalation of breath from the lungs," says Dr. Robin Dunbar, a professor of evolutionary psychology at Oxford. "The muscles of the diaphragm have to work very hard." We've all heard the phrase "laugh until it hurts," he points out. Prolonged laughing can be painful and exhausting.

The cool thing is that Dunbar's 2009 research revealed that like intense exercise, intense laughter increases our pain thresholds. That's right, the same endorphins that are released during intense exercise and help with pain management, are also released after an intense laughing session!

In addition to increasing pain thresholds by releasing endorphins, here are a few other physical benefits of laughter:

- Relaxes the whole body for up to forty-five minutes after a laughing session.
- Boosts the immune system by decreasing stress and increasing antibody-producing immune-cells (called T-cells).
- Protects the heart by improving the function of blood vessels, increasing blood flow, and lowering blood pressure. Research shows that fifteen minutes of laughter per day is equivalent to thirty minutes of cardiovascular exercise.
- Burns the same calories as walking at a slow to moderate pace.
- Improves breathing and can help with respiratory ailments such as asthma.
- Works out your abs, shoulders, and diaphragm.
- Improves sleep quality.
- Everyday take some time to laugh! Your body will thank you!

Cognitive Health

Learn Something New
Commit to learning something new. Take up a new sport, learn to play an instrument, learn a foreign language. Challenge your brain because just like everything else, "if you don't use it, you will lose it."

I will commit to learning_____.

CHAPTER M PREP

1. Begin Chapter M's affirmation. (still to be done looking only at your eyes, repeating seven times, morning and night)
   My body is nourished and healthy.
2. Foam roll daily and before workouts. Do only the corrective exercises that are still difficult for you. After foam rolling, use a dynamic warmup before beginning your workout.
3. By now, recognizing and handling distress, this should be automatic. Continue to find healthy ways to turn times of distress into times of eustress.
4. How are your eating patterns going? Are you at four hours between meals and a twelve-hour fast between dinner and breakfast? (Remember if you are diabetic, you are to clear all modifications with your doctor.)
5. Continue to use the hypnosis video to work on revealing afflictions and receiving affirmations. The goal is to be able to self-hypnotize and to use anchors to drive behavior and thought until they become habit. Record your progress here:

   _____

   _____

6. Continue using the journal format that is best for you. What have you noticed so far? Has anything changed for you?

   _____

   _____

7. Did you try a vegetable juice? What did you think?

8. Have you gotten the hang of juggling? If not, keep at it!

9. Continue to bless others with acts of kindness anytime you can!

10. Speaking others' love languages can change the dynamics of even the toughest relationships. How are you using this new tool?

11. Laugh daily!

⌐ CHAPTER M ⌐

Emotional Health

Myers Briggs Personality Test

This information is a direct quote from www.myersbriggs.org.

The purpose of the Myers-Briggs Type Indicator® (MBTI®) personality inventory is to make the theory of psychological types described by C.G. Jung understandable and useful in people's lives. The essence of the theory is that much seemingly random variation in the behavior is actually quite orderly and consistent, being due to basic differences in the way individuals prefer to use their perception and judgment.

"Perception involves all the ways of becoming aware of things, people, happenings, or ideas. Judgment involves all the ways of coming to conclusions about what has been perceived. If people differ systematically in what they perceive and in how they reach conclusions, then it is only reasonable for them to differ correspondingly in their interests, reactions, values, motivations, and skills."

In developing the Myers-Briggs Type Indicator [instrument], the aim of Isabel Briggs Myers, and her mother, Katharine Briggs, was to make the insights of type theory accessible to individuals and groups. They addressed the two related goals in the developments and application of the MBTI instrument:

1. The identification of basic preferences of each of the four dichotomies specified or implicit in Jung's theory.
2. The identification and description of the sixteen distinctive personality types that result from the interactions among the preferences.

Favorite world: Do you prefer to focus on the outer world or on your own inner world? This is called Extraversion (E) or Introversion (I).

Information: Do you prefer to focus on the basic information you take in or do you prefer to interpret and add meaning? This is called Sensing (S) or Intuition (N).

Decisions: When making decisions, do you prefer to first look at logic and consistency or first look at the people and special circumstances? This is called Thinking (T) or Feeling (F).

Structure: In dealing with the outside world, do you prefer to get things decided or do you prefer to stay open to new information and options? This is called Judging (J) or Perceiving (P).

Your Personality Type: When you decide on your preference in each category, you have your own personality type, which can be expressed as a code with four letters.

Take the test on their website or if you know your type you can get more information about the sixteen different types as well. There are three ways to take the test. If you just want the info without a consultation, go to mbtionline.com.

This is a fun personality test and is just one more way to understand yourself and others better.

I am an INTJ, which surprises many people because I appear to be very outgoing and gregarious. And my test actually says, "Slightly more introverted" so I do love people and being around people and having a good time, but I recharge alone. That is one of the major differences with an "I" versus an "E." A true extrovert recharges by being surrounded by others whereas a true introvert must recharge alone and can feel overwhelmed and exhausted after too much social interaction.

Nutritional Health

Macro-nutrients and Micro-nutrients

Check out www.rhondahuff.com for the video lesson, "Chapter M"

What's the big deal? Food is food, right? Well…not exactly…and here's why.

What is food? It is defined as any nutritious substance that people or animals eat or drink, or that plants absorb, in order to maintain life and growth.

But what exactly are these substances? Well they can be broken down into macro- and micro-nutrients. Here's the difference:

Macro-nutrients are the substances required in relatively large amounts by living organisms and micro-nutrients are the substances required in trace amounts by living organisms.

Macronutrients are the structural and energy-giving caloric components of our foods—carbohydrates, fats and proteins.

Micronutrients are the vitamins, minerals, trace elements, phytochemicals, and antioxidants that are **essential** for good health.

Begin SOAPBOX…

Often people will ignore micronutrients because they think that because our bodies require "trace" amounts, they are unimportant. And in an ideal world, this may be the case. But in the industrialized world, it isn't that simple.

Here is one of the most common things I hear as a health practitioner: "I just have no energy. I eat well. I use the—fill in the blank with the diet trend of the week—way of eating but around 3 p.m. I crash and by 9 p.m. I have eaten a pantry full of carbs. Nothing works for me."

"Nothing" is no thing, right? And it is correct that no thing will ever work, at least not for long. It takes "a lot of things." But "a lot of things" doesn't have to be synonymous with hard things. Think about it. How many diets have you tried? How many were you willing to do for the rest of your life? I have yet to meet a single person who could say to me with 100 percent resolve that they had found a diet that they were willing to follow until death do they part. So why do we continue to spend hundreds of dollars buying the program, throwing away all of our food, re-buying the "right" foods, and suffering every day because we just freaking want a hamburger? Yeah…

Well, if you have a simple understanding of macro- and micro-nutrients, you will never have to diet again. Here is a list of "a lot of simple things" that are essential to never having to diet again. Don't make them hard. And stop being stubborn, trying to convince yourself that it makes no difference where the food comes from. Pay now or pay later. It's your choice.

End SOAPBOX.

A Lot of Simple Things:

1. Processed foods are essentially devoid of nutrients.

    a. Processing strips the foods of many of its vitamins, minerals, and phytochemicals in order to give the food a longer shelf life.

    b. Micronutrients are damaged by heat, air, water, and fat. But not each are damaged by all. A good general rule is to limit the amount of time you allow your foods to be exposed to these elements.

        i.   Cooking with water? Use as little as possible. Can it be lightly steamed instead?

        ii. Cooking in oil? Use as little as possible and cook thoroughly but don't overcook.

        iii. Eating leftovers? Every day it loses potency. After two days, it has lost about 50 percent of its micronutrient content. Leftovers can also lead to inflammation in the body!

        iv. Blending your vegetables? Choose equipment without high centrifugal forces.

2. Animals fed unadulterated foods that are their natural food sources have thousands more micronutrients and cause less allergic reactions.

    a. Farm-raised salmon is colored pink and fed diets of corn and soy—most of which is genetically modified—chicken/feather meal, artificial coloring, and synthetic astaxanthin, which is not approved for human consumption. And thanks to these unnatural fish foods, the healthy Omega-3 fats are less than 50 percent of what they would be in salmon caught out in the wild. You eat what they ate!

    b. Factory-raised chickens are given a chlorine bath to kill pathogens and this chlorine makes its way into you. Chlorine is toxic to your thyroid.

    c. Grass-fed beef is high in CLA, which helps us handle stress better. It is not found in grain-fed beef.

    d. Grain-fed beef is more likely to harbor E-coli. A cow cannot digest grain. For more information about that, watch the 2008 documentary, "Food, Inc."

3. Organic produce is simply safer. It's not that it necessarily has more nutrients—the soil it is grown in determines that—but it is less toxic to your liver function.

    a. And just a thought…if insects are smart enough to not eat pesticide-laden foods yet we eat them, how smart does that make us?

4. Local produce that is grown without chemicals and is grown on healthy, rotated soil is much higher in nutrients than any other produce.
5. So, to repeat the FOOD© acronym from Chapter F:
   a. Free of anti-nutrients. It's all about the ingredients.
   b. Organic when possible
   c. Original in form. And in what the animal would naturally eat.
   d. Dense in nutrients. The most nutrients come from great, clean, rotated soil.

You see, it's not just following a diet. Diets will fail you every single time unless you are bound to them until death. Eat real food, practice balance and moderation, and remember to ask yourself "will this make me gain or lose health?"

Physical Health

Make-up and Skincare

As with food, try to steer away from chemicals in your personal care products. It only takes twenty-six seconds for some chemicals placed on the skin to enter the bloodstream. Of course, our skin itself is a barrier and some molecules are too big to actually enter the bloodstream via the skin. Some products are designed to stay on the top layer of the skin. It is still a concern, however, when you read that a baby is often born with over 200 toxic chemicals already in his or her bloodstream. A little prudence can be a good thing.

To keep things simple, I am not providing an exhaustive list. I am mostly following the Environmental Working Group recommendations (check out http://www.ewg.org/skindeep/). I encourage you to do your own research, as there are many others. If you are pregnant or have small children, be especially diligent in providing the safest possible products for your young ones.

The brands listed are drugstore brands, and remember, there are many more, including many more-expensive brands out there. Once again, just trying to keep it simple.

Product Type	AVOID	USE
Hair Care	Chemical hair straighteners Coal tar hair dye Dark permanent hair dyes Lead Parabens Phthalates Quaternium-15 Resorcinol	ACURE Organics Mineral Fusion Pacifica Beauty SheaMoisture
Hand Sanitizers	Ethanol Ethyl alcohol (in at least 60 percent alcohol) Triclosan	
Fragrance	BHA	
Nails	Dibutyl phthalate (DBP) Formaldehyde Formalin Toulene Pregnant? Skip polish	Mineral Fusion
Skin/Lip	Alpha hydroxy acids (lactic acid) Beta hydroxy acids (glycolic acid) Boric acid Bronopol DEA (diethanolamine), MEA (Monoethanolamine) & TEA (triethanolamine) Hydroquinone Parabens PEG/ceteareth/polyethylene Petrloleum distillates Phthalates Quaternium-15 Retinoic acid Retinol in daytime products Retinyl acetate Retinyl palmitate Sodium Borate	ACURE Organics Dr. Bronner's Eco-Tools (makeup brushes) Mineral Fusion Pacifica Beauty SheaMoisture S.W. Basics

Soap	Parabens	Dr. Bronner's
	Phthalates	Pacifica Beauty
	Triclocarban	SheaMoisture
	Triclosan	
Sunscreen	Added insect repellent	Hats/shade in mid-day
	Aerosol spray	Spf 15 to 50
	Oxybenzone	Titanium dioxide avobenzone
	Powder sunscreen	(3 percent)
	Retinyl palmitate	Zinc oxide
	SPF above 50	Use a lot and reapply
		frequently
Toothpaste	Triclosan	

Cognitive Health

Map It!

Take several minutes to study a map of the USA. Then recreate the map by drawing a full USA map with all the states from memory.

If this was easy, try other continents or the whole world!

CHAPTER N PREP

1. Begin Chapter N's affirmation. (still to be done looking only at your eyes, repeating seven times, morning and night)
   I choose to see the positive things around me.
2. Foam roll daily and before workouts. Do only the corrective exercises that are still difficult for you. After foam rolling, use a dynamic warmup before beginning your workout.
3. After nine weeks, eating patterns should be regular, at least four hours apart, and waiting twelve-hours between dinner and breakfast. You are ideally eating three smart meals per day and rarely or never snacking between. (Remember if you are diabetic, you are to clear all modifications with your doctor.) If this is not the case, determine how much effort you have put into this or if this is simply not a negotiable area in your life. Either is ok. It's ultimately your choice.
4. Continue using the journal format that is best for you. What have you noticed so far? Has anything changed for you?

   _____

   _____

5. Has vegetable juicing become a regular practice for you? What changes have you noticed?

   _____

   _____

6. Have you gotten the hang of juggling? If not, keep at it!
7. Continue to bless others with acts of kindness anytime you can!
8. Speaking the love languages of others can change the dynamics of even the toughest relationships. How are you using this new tool?
9. Laugh daily!
10. Get your macro- and micro-nutrients each day through wholesome and healthy foods.
11. Continue to make small changes in cleaning up your skincare and makeup products.

CHAPTER N

Emotional Health

Negativity

Negativity is defined as *"the expression of criticism of or pessimism about something."* Some people believe that negativity should never be a part of us. I say this is hogwash. If we are going to live authentically healthy lives, the pendulum must always include a sense of balance. The pendulum can't stay stuck on one side.

Another theory I like to question is the "glass half empty" versus "glass half full" person. Well, if I am being authentic, then sometimes my glass is half full and sometimes it is half empty. Sometimes it is running over, and other times it is dry as a bone!

The one question I have is...

What are you known for?

Would your closest friends and family say you are usually a negative person or that you are usually a positive person? No one can be characterized as "always negative" or "always positive." It isn't possible. People who don't know me well will say about me, "She is always so positive!" My closest friends and family, however, would say something closer to, "She is a human with human emotions, and yet she tries hard to make the best out of situations." I am mostly known for being positive. And for many years, I would venture to say that except for one or two people in my life, I faked that

I was "always" positive. I wasn't living authentically. I couldn't risk people knowing my weaknesses. I wasn't confident enough to believe people would still love me if they saw the real me. It was only when I became bold enough to be authentic that I could share the real me. And then something really cool happened, people loved me anyway.

If you are known for "always being positive," ask yourself if you are living authentically. And if you aren't, get curious about it.

If you are known for "always being negative," ask yourself what is behind the negativity. It can be a trait that is passed down generationally, pops up as a protective mechanism, evolved as a form of self-sabotage, or even a habit that simply took hold at some point in your life and now controls you.

And if you are known for usually being positive and trying to make the best of things, then hallelujah! Keep spreading the authentically positive vibes. The world needs you!

Nutritional Health

Nutritional Deficiencies

Believe it or not, malnutrition is rampant in this country. How can a country with 74 percent of its population being obese be starving to death? Well, there are two basic reasons, one of which we have full control over.

1. Eating too many processed, dead, or chemical-laden foods. The more processed the food, the less nutritious the food becomes. This goes back to the FOOD© from Chapter F: *Free of anti-nutrients.* If the ingredient list has more than five ingredients and you can't pronounce them, don't eat it. It is devoid of nutrients even if it says "fortified." *Organic when possible.* Steering clear of pesticides/herbicides. *Original in Form.* Eating as close to the food's original state as possible. *Dense in Nutrients.* Eating foods that give the most nutritional bang for their buck.

2. Nutrient-depleted soil. In 1950, an apple had 4.3 mg of iron. Today that same apple has .18 mg of iron. We would have to eat twenty-six apples to get the same amount of iron now as then. And we wonder why so many people are anemic? We have little control over this. The key is to fight back. Encourage your local farmers to rotate crops and let the fields rest every seven years (and give them the tips listed after the timeline below). Then support them financially by buying form them so they can continue to do the right

thing. Support legislation that is for US not for BIG AGRA. August Dunning gives this timeline:

1925: Mechanized farming began; depleting minerals faster than microorganisms in the soil could replenish them, which were needed for the following year's growth.

1946: The introduction of ammonium nitrate fertilizer stimulated greater yields, but also changed the chemistry of the soil structure. This bound up calcium, burned out the Humus, and caused acidic conditions, leading to the formation of gasses like formaldehyde and alcohol, which attracted pests.

1950s: Pesticides were introduced to correct the new pest problem. This could have been fixed by replenishing the mineral content to fix the pH and re-establish microorganism/mineral balance. Pesticides also kill microorganisms and thus nature's ability to provide ionic elements needed for proper plant growth and nutrition was further destroyed.

1990s: Genetically engineered (GE) seeds and glyphosate were introduced— now any minerals left were hyper-chelated and made unavailable to plants. Now we have produce that has been engineered to keep away pests (once again—INSTEAD of rotating and resting to replenish the soil). So now the glyphosate formulation (POEA) is in the fruit itself as opposed to being sprayed with it. And we must ask, what is the correlation between the loss of minerals and the addition of "round-up" to the huge increase in disease that we saw happen around the same time?

August Dunning also recommends the following steps to replenish the soil:

1. Add naturally-occurring ocean minerals back to the soil.
2. Have earthworms in your gardens and fields.
3. Use *Biochar.*
4. Check out www.ecoorganics.com for more info.

What can you do personally to help our children's and grandchildren's years be healthier? We can all do something, even if it is writing an email to our senators. One voice is like 1,000. I learned that while leading a Youth Advocacy Group. When one person takes the time to write or call, it is counted as 1,000 as the statistics show that when one person speaks up, about 1,000 more feel the same way but will not speak up. We must be our own advocates! Let's speak up!

Resources on finding non-GMO foods:

- Eat Well Guide (United States & Canada)
- Farm Match (United States)
- Local Harvest (United States)
- Weston A. Price Foundation (United States)
- Organic Food Directory (Australia)
- Eat Wild (Canada)
- Organic Explorer (New Zealand)

Physical Health

No Equipment Required

Check out www.rhondahuff.com for the video lesson, "Chapter N"

Sometimes you just don't have time to get to the gym. That is the beauty of bodyweight exercises. In this video lesson, we will show you a few more exercises that require no equipment and how to modify them if needed. We will follow the same format that you learned in Chapter I. Hopefully you have a good handle on how to follow this type of plan now.

Cognitive Health

Nondominance Exercise

Switch it up!

For the next seven days, use your nondominant body part! Brush your teeth with your nondominant hand, put your pants on the other leg first, put the opposite shoe on first, carry your purse on the opposite side of the body, practice writing with the nondominant hand, eat with your nondominant hand. You get the picture. It's harder than you think. But oh so good for your brain!

CHAPTER O PREP

1. Begin Chapter O's affirmation. (still to be done looking only at your eyes, repeating seven times, morning and night)
    I am bold enough to own up to my mistakes.
2. Foam roll daily and before workouts. Do only the corrective exercises that are still difficult for you. After foam rolling, use a dynamic warmup before beginning your workout.
3. Revisit the Four Agreements in Chapter F. Yes it is that important. We all need these reminders.
4. The FOOD© principle and knowing what foods you enjoy that are supplying prebiotics and probiotics should now be habit. Journey on with this incredibly healthy habit!
5. Have you gotten the hang of juggling? If not, keep at it!
6. Continue to bless others with acts of kindness anytime you can!
7. Speaking the love languages of others can change the dynamics of even the toughest relationships. How are you using this new tool?
8. Laugh daily!
9. Get your macro- and micro-nutrients each day through wholesome and healthy foods.
10. Continue to make small changes in cleaning up your skincare and makeup products.

11. Continue to keep a check on negativity.
12. Work on your brain health by doing more and more things with your non-dominant side.

CHAPTER O

Emotional Health

Owning Up

Mistakes. We all make them. We know that everyone makes mistakes and that no one is perfect and yet our instinct is usually to cover them up, blame someone else, or blatantly deny them. Why can it be so hard to admit when we make a mistake? The answer is probably different for each of us but probably all has its root in one thing—FEAR, defined as *an anxious feeling, caused by our anticipation of some imagined event or experience.*

Fear of being found inadequate

Fear of getting in trouble

Fear of being vulnerable

Fear of humiliation or shame (aka ego-death)

Fear of insults and criticisms

Fear of not being able to make it right

Fear of rejection

Fear of (fill in the blank)_____

However, if we dare to step up in boldness and admit our mistakes, a few incredible things happen!

1. We learn something and are less likely to make the same mistake next time. We actually learn more from mistakes and failures than we do from successes.

2. If we quickly own up to our mistakes and authentically seek to make them right, they are less likely to turn into even bigger problems.

3. We gain the respect of others. That's right, most people actually respect those who have the boldness to own up to mistakes. Of course, there always will be those few who belittle us and hold our mistakes against us. The question then becomes, "how much power am I going to allow this person to have over me?" Maybe the relationship needs to be reevaluated.

4. It helps us to stop using global labels with others. When we realize mistakes often happen due to circumstances and not character, we can have more compassion for the mistakes of others. For example, if you miss someone's birthday, it is probably because you had a busy week or stressful things on your mind, right? How often has someone missed your birthday and you immediately assumed it was because they were self-centered? That's using a global label, and it attacks character. Admitting our own mistakes allows us to experience both from others. They either understand the circumstance or they attack our character. That, my friends, leads quickly to empathy. And empathy is a great thing!

5. We learn to take responsibility for our lives. We begin to more accurately see who we are and how our choices affect others. The opposite of this is the victim mentality—thinking that things are always happening TO us, instead of us actually realizing that we have quite a bit of control over our own lives. For example, if you are chronically late for work and you look for "legitimate" reasons—"I hit every red light this morning," "My dog took forever going potty," "I had to be behind Granny Slowpokes AGAIN today"—you will never take responsibility for the fact that maybe you shouldn't have had that second cup of coffee or that you should have gotten up fifteen minutes earlier. And yes, the best-laid plans can at times fail but more often than not, it boils down to our own personal choices.

This week pay close attention to opportunities to "own up." It just may change your life in a way that enriches your character and enhances the lives of those around you.

Nutritional Health

Orange

I love the color orange! According to researchers who study the psychological effects of color, the lively color of orange represents strength and endurance and can promote a bright and energizing mood.

Those benefits are found through orange foods as well. The orange hue in fruits and vegetables is due to the antioxidant beta-carotene (Vitamin A). Other important nutrients found in orange fruits and vegetables include zeaxanthin, flavonoids, lycopene, potassium, and vitamin C. All these nutrients work together to support healthy skin, hair, and vision, increase immunity, decrease risk of cancer, and support a healthy heart.

Here are a few to check out.

Pumpkins, apricots, cantaloupe, carrots, mangoes, oranges, sweet potatoes, peaches, orange bell peppers, nectarines, tangerines

This week, make an effort to eat at least one serving of orange foods every day!

Physical Health

Outdoor Activities

Try to spend time outdoors this week. I am actually writing this chapter's module outside, and it is so relaxing and energizing!

The benefits of regularly enjoying nature are abundant. Here are just a few to motivate you to get outside:

Vitamin D (which is technically a hormone, not a vitamin)
Ten to fifteen minutes a day, without sunscreen, may boost your Vitamin D production

Eye health
Prevent Computer Vision Syndrome (CVS): symptoms include blurred vision, double vision, dry/red eyes, eye irritation, headaches, and neck or back pain. Get outside and enjoy looking into the distance. Nature wants to share its beauty.

Artificial light provokes nearsightedness: A 2007 Ohio University study found that American children with two myopic parents were four times less likely to be nearsighted if they spent at least two hours per day outside than those who were outside less than an hour a day. Artificial light is a problem; natural light may be the solution.

Better sleep

Too much time inside throws off the circadian rhythms in the body, which help regulate our sleep cycles.

"Fresh Air"

Outdoor pollution is bad for your health but INDOOR pollution is far worse! The California Air Resources Board says, "indoor air-pollutants are 25 percent to 62 percent greater than outside levels, and this difference poses a serious risk to health." Some of these health risks are heart disease, lung cancer, chronic bronchitis, and asthma attacks.

Grounding/Earthing

This practice reminds me of warm summer days lying on the grass with my mom and sister and making objects out of the clouds above us. The theory of Grounding (or Earthing) states that because the earth is negatively charged—and has a greater negative charge than your body—we absorb earth's electrons. The rubber soles of our shoes prevent this absorption of electrons from occurring. Research so far is finding that this practice has an intense anti-inflammatory and energizing effect on the body. So, get your skin in contact with the earth. Just another reason to head to the beach, right?

Exercise

Take your exercise routine outside.

Healthy Psyche

Being in nature provides improvements in attention span, boosts in serotonin levels—the feel-good neurotransmitter—triggers creativity, and shows increased activity in parts of the brain responsible for love, empathy, and emotional stability.

Go outside and enjoy the beauty of nature.

Cognitive Health

Occupational Inventory

Check out www.rhondahuff.com for the video lesson, "Chapter O"

One thing I have noticed when working one-on-one with health coaching clients is that people forget how great they are. They forget the skills, gifts, and talents that have led to life accomplishments. This is so unfortunate as the world needs our lights to shine. When our lights shine, it gives others permission to do the same.

I am not speaking of a prideful or boastful assessment of ourselves. I am speaking of an inventory that is **led by meekness and humility but never stops short of extraordinary**. San Diego pastor and author, Dr. David Jeremiah, has a definition of meekness that I love: "Power under control." It is not failing to go where you need to go but not going further than is needed.

Take some time to do an occupational inventory. This is like an extended resume. Start as early in your life as you can remember. Your occupation as a kid may simply have been to be a kid. Maybe you had chores, perhaps you played on recreational teams, or perhaps you babysat your siblings. Whatever you did, consider what you did well and write it down below. Were you the best runner on your team? Why? Were you the best table-setter in your family? Why? Did you discover a way to do something that was better than anyone else in your class? How?

What aspects of your personality, strengths, and character made you great? Write every single thing down, even if it seems minor.

Once it is all written down, read it, slowly. WOW! You are amazing. More amazing than you ever realized, right? You are you! You are special! You were created for a purpose. Do you see it? Can you feel it? Be bold enough to own it!

I know this exercise will be hard for some of you. I know you will pick apart everything you have ever done and try hard to minimize or mock it. Go back and do the hypnosis activities again. Get curious! Work it out and work it through. Don't stop until you have an occupational inventory that depicts the wonderfully created human being that you are!

My Occupational Inventory

_____

_____

_____

_____

_____

CHAPTER P PREP

1. Begin Chapter P's affirmation. (still to be done looking only at your eyes, repeating seven times, morning and night)
   I am at peace.
2. Foam roll daily and before workouts. Do only the corrective exercises that are still difficult for you. After foam rolling, use a dynamic warmup before beginning your workout.
3. Continue to bless others with acts of kindness anytime you can!
4. Speaking others' love languages can change the dynamics of even the toughest relationships. How are you using this new tool?
5. Laugh daily!
6. Get your macro- and micro-nutrients each day through wholesome and healthy foods.
7. Continue to research and learn about healthier makeup and skincare products.
8. Are you being more positive? Like authentically positive? If so, it feels great doesn't it?
9. Own up to your mistakes.
10. Get outside and enjoy nature!
11. Take one more look at your Occupational Inventory. Now smile because you are awesome!

CHAPTER P

Emotional Health

Peacefulness

Peacefulness is an inner sense of calm. Even adventure-seeking people like myself still seek to have an inner sense of calm. I love being on the go, learning new things, and experiencing crazy adventures. But even so, I need peace. I crave peace. I desire peace. And I have peace.

Obviously finding peace will be different for each of us. People find peace through prayer, meditation, journaling, quietness, etc. Have you discovered a way to experience peace? If so, write it below:

_____

_____

_____

_____

If not, get curious. What is at the root of not being able to find peace? The answer may quickly flood your mind or it may take some real work to discover. Allow your subconscious to share some insights with you. Do a short self-hypnosis session if needed.

Share your thoughts here and decide on a plan for bringing peacefulness into your daily life:

_____

_____

_____

Nutritional Health

Psychology of Food

Check out www.rhondahuff.com for the video lesson, "Chapter P"

Did you know that the attitude with which you eat food affects how your body metabolizes it?

Here is an example of the power of the mind: In 1983, medical researchers tested a new chemotherapy drug. One group of cancer patients received the actual drug being tested while another group received a placebo, a harmless saltwater substance. Of the cancer patients receiving the real chemotherapy 74 percent lost their hair. But remarkably, so did 31 percent of the placebo group. Such is the power of the mind. The only reason the patients on the placebo lost their hair was because they believed they would.

Another interesting study shows that people who were given a placebo but told it was Vitamin C had significantly fewer colds than the people who were given the real Vitamin C but were told it was a placebo.

Here is the science behind what the mind/body connection does when you are getting ready to eat food.

1. The thought/image of a food occurs in the cerebral cortex.
2. This info is relayed electrochemically to the limbic system, which regulates emotions and physiological functions such as hunger, thirst, temperature, sex drive, heart rate, and blood pressure.
   a. Within the limbic system is the hypothalamus, which integrates the activities of the mind with the biology of the body.
   b. When you look at a food with delight and consume it with a peaceful and grateful attitude, the hypothalamus sends signals to the salivary glands, esophagus, stomach, intestines, pancreas, liver, and gallbladder via the

parasympathetic nervous system. Digestion is stimulated and you'll have a full, healthy metabolic breakdown of the food while burning its calories more efficiently.

c. When you look at a food with contempt and consume it with guilt or fear of it making you fat, the hypothalamus sends signals to the salivary glands, esophagus, stomach, intestines, pancreas, liver, and gallbladder via the sympathetic nervous system. Digestion is inhibited, which means you'll be eating your food but not fully metabolizing it. It may stay in your digestive system longer, which can diminish your population of healthy gut bacteria, increase the release of toxic by-products into the bloodstream, decrease your calorie-burning efficiency via increased insulin and cortisol, which would cause you to store more of your food as body fat.

So, the thoughts you think about the food you eat instantly become reality in your body via the central nervous system. Do you get this? This is incredible. It certainly doesn't mean that we should eat all the junk we want with a happy heart and not worry about it. But it does once again point to the importance of balance. To be healthy we need to eat healthy, energy-dense foods. However, balance also means that on that rare occasion that you get a hankering for ice cream, eat it! And enjoy it with happiness and gratitude. The important thing here is to choose REAL ice cream! The ingredient list should look something like this: *organic milk, organic cream, organic evaporated cane juice, organic egg yolks, organic nonfat milk, organic vanilla extract* (Three Twins Madagascar Vanilla). Don't eat the crap with several nasty ingredients. Go for full fat, real food. Less is more as it will satisfy you more quickly and your body knows what to do with real food.

Physical Health

Pain Management
Pain is the number one reason Americans go to the doctor. In 2013 there were 207 million prescriptions written for pain killers (compared to 76 million in 1991). There are many reasons why using pain medication is risky but the issue I want to discuss today is that they only cover symptoms and do not cure anything. Therefore, you are doomed to a life on pain killers unless you can figure out the problem and act to solve the problem.

You have already been working toward this through the foam rolling and corrective exercises. Below is a list of other alternative treatments to consider when dealing with pain.

1. **Acupuncture:** Recognized as an effective treatment for pain by the World Health Organization, acupuncture is an ancient Chinese healing art that has been in use for over 2,000 years. The practice involves inserting hair-thin needles into various points on the skin to regulate movement within the body's meridian system.

2. **Aromatherapy;** This treatment uses scents from essential plant oils that are applied to the skin and/or inhaled. This treatment dates back thousands of years and research has proven that it is effective for decreasing pain symptoms in people with rheumatoid arthritis, headaches, and cancer.

3. **Biofeedback:** Teaches the patient to consciously affect normally involuntary bodily functions, such as heart rate, muscle tension, and blood pressure. An electromyography device (EMG) can be used to measure muscle tension but has been found to be among the most useless feedback systems for chronic pain.

4. **Chiropractic:** Chiropractic has been shown to be effective for a variety of pain syndromes, including lower back pain, neck pain, carpal tunnel, headaches, and sports injuries.

5. **Frequency Specific Microcurrent:** Offers exciting promise in working with tissues unresponsive to conventional efforts such as nerve pain, nerve damage nerve injury, scar tissue, adhesions, inflammation, and the ability to facilitate healing of acute and chronic injuries. It is also used as a supportive treatment for chronic conditions like chronic Lyme disease, CFS, and fibromyalgia. The frequencies appear to change a variety of conditions and tissues, alleviating pain and function in a large number of clinical conditions.

6. **Hypnotherapy**—hypnotherapy produces relaxation and induces an altered state of consciousness, which has been shown to help people gain control over their states of awareness, which can in turn help them gain control over their physical body, including their pain symptoms. Research suggests that hypnosis can help reduce the need for pain medication by decreasing the anxiety that's typically associated with pain.

7. **Massage**—by influencing the muscles, circulation, lymphatic system, and nervous system, massage is a time-tested healing method for all types of pain.

8. **Movement**—joints that are stiff, achy and sluggish crave movement. For years we were taught to rest achy joints but research now shows that what we really need is movement. Work toward full ranges of motion in all joints.

9. **Relaxation Therapy:** Pain causes stress, which causes more pain, which causes more stress, which causes more pain. It is an endless cycle. When there is pain, the body goes into a fight or flight situation and blood pressure will elevate and muscles will tense. This just exacerbates the pain. Common relaxation techniques that are proven to reduce pain symptoms are guided imagery, progressive muscle relaxation, meditation, and tai chi.

10. **Trigger Point Therapy:** Alleviates the source of pain through cycles of isolated pressure and release. A trigger point is a contracture—not a spasm—within muscle tissue that causes pain in other parts of the body. For example, a trigger point in the quads may produce referral pain in the knee. You can experience a significant decrease in pain after just one treatment.

If you struggle with pain, become your own advocate. Listen to your body. Get curious about your pain. Find solutions not band-aids.

Cognitive Health

Poetry

Poetry; the literary work in which special intensity is given to the expression of feelings and ideas by the use of distinctive style and rhythm.

When was the last time you read—or wrote—poetry?

Reading poetry is fantastic for the brain. Studies show that reading poetry:

- stimulates the right hemisphere of the brain
- produces more activity in the regions of the brain that are linked to memory than any other type of reading
- activates certain areas of the brain, such as the posterior cingulate cortex and the medial temporal lobes, which have been linked to introspection (the ability to examine your own mental and emotional processes).
- In addition to the benefits of reading poetry, writing poetry also has remarkable virtues:
- helps emotional regulation

- when we express ourselves through writing, we are able to subconsciously regulate our levels of anxiety, fear, and sadness
- calms down the brain
- restores a sense of mental balance

Make a commitment to do two things:

1. Read one poem each day this week.
2. Write one poem during the week. Record below:

_____

_____

_____

_____

_____

_____

_____

_____

_____

_____

_____

_____

_____

_____

_____

_____

_____

CHAPTER Q PREP

1. Begin Chapter Q's affirmation. (You know what to do…)
    I look for the quality of interactions in my life.
2. Foam roll daily and before workouts. Do only the corrective exercises that are still difficult for you. After foam rolling, use a dynamic warmup before beginning your workout.
3. Continue to bless others with acts of kindness anytime you can!
4. Continue to explore your own and your loved ones' love language.
5. Laugh daily!
6. Get your macro- and micro-nutrients each day through wholesome and healthy foods.
7. Continue to keep a check on negativity.
8. Own up to your mistakes.
9. Get outside and enjoy nature. While you are there, practice peacefulness.
10. Eat your food with a grateful heart.
11. Continue to experiment with healthy ways to deal with pain. The body is amazing in its ability to self-heal.
12. Get creative again and write another poem. You can do it! Make it silly or serious. It doesn't matter to your brain. It just craves creativity.

CHAPTER Q

Emotional Health

Quiet Time

Quiet time and peacefulness tend to go hand in hand. If you have been working on your state of peacefulness from last week you may have instituted some quiet time into your schedule.

Quiet time is uncomfortable to many people because they find it hard to deal with silence and stillness. I can totally relate! The first time I tried to do a restorative yoga session I thought I was going to lose my mind. There seemed to be "so many other important things I should be doing with my time." That, my friends, is a lie straight outta hell.

As a society we must stop making status symbols out of "busyness" and "stressed-out." Being busy and stressed out makes us less healthy and less effective. Why has the need for people to think we are busy and stressed become so important to us? Let's recognize how terrible this is and work to shift this perspective. I am not so important that the world will stop spinning if I take some time to nurture ME. That's right, it is OK for us to take care of ourselves. It is healthy and necessary if we want to be more effective at helping others.

Take a few moments to quiz yourself on this. Do you constantly tell people how busy or stressed you are? Be honest. Ask your spouse or a close friend. I believe that sometimes we are in such a habit of doing this that we don't recognize it as being a constant occurrence.

What did you discover?

_____

_____

_____

Make a covenant with yourself to stop this. Write a plan of how to keep yourself accountable.

Nutritional Health

Quarter your plate

Visualize your plate. Divide the plate into four sections.

One section is for protein.

One section is for green vegetables (preferably leafy).

One section is for colorful vegetables (remember to eat the rainbow).

One section is for a starchy vegetable OR a grain OR fruit OR, on occasion, a small dessert. Notice I used the word "or" here. It is one of the four, not all of them.

Add brain healthy fats, such as avocado, coconut oil, olive oil, nuts, and seeds within the other sections. And of course remember that if you are trying to lose weight, nuts and seeds are high in calories so just be aware of that.

Physical Health

Quality over Quantity

Check out www.rhondahuff.com for the video lesson, "Chapter Q"

I see lots of workout videos online that make me cringe. The positions some of these workouts put your bodies in are very dangerous. Many of these effects aren't acute injuries but things that crop up months or years later.

Workouts that use quick, explosive movements and AREN'T supervised properly are flat out dangerous. Think quality of movement. As with the correctives you began in Chapter C, form is everything. Improper form not only leads to an increased risk of injury, it also prevents the very results you are working so hard to attain.

In today's video I will cover some of the most common form foibles that I have seen over the years.

Whatever form of exercise you choose, perfect the movements first. Slow down and really learn how to do it perfectly. Remember that practice makes permanent, only perfect practice makes perfect. There is no need for permanent pain, recurring pain, or even momentary pain when focusing on the quality of the movement can prevent all three.

Cognitive Health

Question Everything

As we have discussed before, neuroplasticity happens throughout life. Our brains change, and we can make choices that allow for that change to be positive or negative. As with other areas of our bodies, the philosophy that "if you don't use it, you lose it" is true for our brains.

This week exercise your brain by asking those weird, crazy, complex questions that may have perplexed you as you grew up or even now. I have always been a "why" person. My parents tell stories of how I exhausted them because I wanted to know the why behind everything. (To their delight, my first child repaid me.)

That inquisitiveness has played well for me as I spend my life asking why: "Why do the hamstrings of MS patients not fire properly regardless of where the lesions are?" "Why don't diets work long-term? "Why can someone with Parkinson's not walk a straight line but can dance like there's no tomorrow? "What must be done to prevent or reverse disease, not just cover up the symptoms of disease?" And I could go on and on. My questions drive my research and my research makes life better for other people.

What are your questions? Ask, research, and learn. Then share it with someone. If you teach it, you've learned it, and if you've learned it, your brain is positively affected.

CHAPTER R PREP

1. Take a step back and just remind yourself of this.
   I fully love and accept myself just as I am right now.
2. Do you? You should! You are wonderful!
3. Begin Chapter R's affirmation (where are your eyes?)
4. I choose to respond, not react, to situations.
5. Foam roll daily and before workouts. Do only the corrective exercises that are still difficult for you. After foam rolling, use a dynamic warmup before beginning your workout.
6. Allow the Four Agreements to help you respond to situations instead of reacting to them.
7. Revisit the hypnosis video if you need a boost.
8. Laugh daily!
9. Get your macro- and micro-nutrients each day through wholesome and healthy foods.
10. Continue to keep a check on negativity.
11. Own up to your mistakes.
12. Get outside and enjoy nature. Take a meditative walk.
13. Eat your food with a grateful heart.
14. Continue to experiment with healthy ways to deal with pain.
15. Take some time to be quiet every day. This can even be done on your meditative walk outside.

CHAPTER R

Emotional Health

Responding Instead of Reacting

We all have heard that we can't control the behavior of others but we can control how we react to it. I would like to take this a step further and suggest that there is a difference between reacting and responding and responding usually results in a better outcome.

When faced with confrontation, a reaction is usually something that happens immediately and without much thought (think knee-jerk reaction). And though our passion about a situation will definitely be made clear in a reaction, it may not bring about the best result.

Responding, on the other hand, involves thoughtful reasoning. It is guided less by emotion (passion) and more by logic. It takes the time needed to cool off and clarify intention before addressing an issue. Here are a few ways to practice the wait before the response.

1. **Stop:** Bite your tongue, pinch your arm, or walk away, but don't allow that first word to slip from your mouth just yet.
2. **Breathe:** Focusing on the breath will calm the sympathetic nervous system and bring awareness to the emotions and feelings arising within, giving you time to control them.

3. **Raise attentiveness:** Become more attentive to what the other person is saying and attempt to understand their viewpoint before voicing your own.

4. **Respond:** Remember to treat others the way you want to be treated. Be respectful.

Nutritional Health

Red / Purple / Blue / Black

Sounds like a really bad bruise, right? But as a bruise is caused by the rupturing of blood vessels, eating these foods will build up the blood, making you healthier, and according to research, slimmer.

Red, purple, blue, and black foods are shown to reduce the risk for high blood pressure, clear free radicals from the blood, reduce inflammation, reduce the buildup of plaque in arteries, and increase HDL—the "happy"—cholesterol). Scientists believe that anthocyanins, compounds that give these foods their color, are responsible for these benefits. And these foods don't stop there. Research is clear that eating these dark foods is cancer-protective and helps prevent diabetes.

Look at your food list and find all the red, purple, blue, and black foods on it. Commit to eating as many of those foods this week as you can. And the ones you love? Add them in to your regular nutrition plan. Your blood—and your waistline—will thank you!

Write your beneficial dark foods here:

_____

_____

_____

_____

Physical Health

Rest and Recovery

To rest is defined as "to cease work or movement in order to relax, refresh oneself, or recover strength."

Recovery is defined as "a return to a normal state of health, mind, or strength." These are things you do to maximize the body's repair. Recovery is multifaceted and encompasses muscle recovery, chemical and hormonal balance, nervous system repair, mental state, and much more.

Both are crucial components of good health and any successful training program, and yet they are the most underutilized. Why? Although I feel there are several layers to this, after working with hundreds of people, I believe the common denominator is our society's emphasis on working harder, pushing further, and climbing that ladder of success. And I am one of the worst offenders. That's right, I struggle with this—hard! And yet I know by watching my own life as well as speaking with others that this is a problem we must address and correct.

Let me be clear, I am NOT saying we should let go of our work ethic. I actually think our work ethic in general in this country could sometimes be much better. Nor am I saying we shouldn't strive for excellence and reach for the top of that ladder. We most definitely should.

What I am saying is that while we are doing this, we need to rest and recover. Constantly "burning the midnight oil" is one of the fastest ways to burn out.

Finding that balance, however, can be incredibly difficult. Our lives are multifaceted, and just because we need to rest and recover doesn't change the fact that after ten hours at work we still have to cook, do laundry, spend quality time with the kids and the spouse, mow the lawn, take three kids to three different practices, oversee homework, prepare for the next day of work, walk the dog, check on family and friends, take a meal to a sick neighbor, plus a myriad of other important things. Makes me want to yell out, "Can I get an Amen?"

Next week we will be looking at some ways to mitigate this. In the meantime, take an inventory of your life this week. Make a list of all the things that must get accomplished in a typical week. Also keep track of the time you rest and recover. I will help you understand these concepts by giving some specific examples.

Rest: sleep, meditation, relaxation, in whatever way that works for you

Recovery: proper hydration, adequate time during and between exercise, nutrition, sunlight, proper posture, self-myofascial release (foam rolling), and stretching.

How much time do you prioritize for rest and recovery? Get serious about this. It can make or break your health.

Weekly to-do list	Weekly rest and recovery

Cognitive Health

Rules of Brain Health

Check out www.rhondahuff.com for the video lesson, "Chapter R"

Brain health is so important that I wanted to review some rules you should follow to ensure a healthy future brain.

- **Find productive ways to deal with stress**. Your brain is built to deal with stress that lasts about thirty seconds. The brain is not designed for long-term stress that leaves you feeling like you have no control. Stress will cause damage to every type of cognitive function: memory, executive function, attention, language skills, thinking skills, and motor skills. It also inhibits your immune system, disrupts your sleep, and causes depression. Are you still working to deal with any distress that creeps into your life?
- **Use it or lose it**. The health of the brain is dependent on brain activity. It is a survival organ designed to solve problems. Keep learning new things.
- **Exercise.** Exercise increases oxygen flow to the brain, which reduces brain-bound free radicals, improving mental sharpness. Exercise also increases the creation of neurons and protects them from damage and stress.
- **Sleep.** As with stress, poor sleep negatively affects cognitive function. Also, it is normal for people to feel a little sleepy around 3 p.m. This may be due to that being about twelve hours past the midpoint of nightly sleep. Try not to make important decisions at 3 p.m.
- **Accept that no two brains are alike (even twins).** Research indicates that there are about 7 billion types of intelligence (the number of people in the world). Everyone has different strengths and weaknesses, and everyone learns in different ways. Instead of making excuses about not liking to read or do puzzles or learn something new, find something (anything) that stimulates your brain. It is essential.
- **Stop multi-tasking**. The human brain cannot multi-task. Repeat that, "The human brain CANNOT multi-task." The brain is a sequential processor and large fractions of a second are consumed every time the brain switches tasks. This is why cellphone talkers are a half-second slower to hit the brakes and get into more accidents. It is also why it is so hard to get back on task after you

have been interrupted. Research is clear that multi-tasking doubles the time it takes to complete a task and leads to 50 percent more errors.

- **Repeat and repeat and repeat.** The brain can only hold about seven pieces of information for up to thirty seconds. Which means that if you want to extend the time information is in your mind, you must repeat that information enough to move it from short-term to long-term storage.
- **Use all of your senses.** They are all important to brain health. Use them.
- **Explore new ideas.** Google takes this power of exploration to heart. Employees are encouraged to spend 20 percent of the workday allowing their mind to go wherever it leads. The proof is in the bottom line: 50 percent of new products, including Gmail and Google News, came from their "20 percent time."

CHAPTER S PREP

1. Begin Chapter S' affirmation.
   I set and respect healthy boundaries.
2. Foam roll daily and before workouts. Do only the corrective exercises that are still difficult for you. After foam rolling, use a dynamic warmup before beginning your workout.
3. Laugh daily!
4. Get your macro- and micro-nutrients each day through wholesome and healthy foods.
5. Continue to keep a check on negativity.
6. Own up to your mistakes.
7. Eat your food mindfully, slowly, chewing thoroughly.
8. Continue to experiment with healthy ways to deal with pain. The body is amazing in its ability to self-heal.
9. Take some time to be quiet every day.
10. Continue to focus on responding not reacting.
11. Work on making red, purple, blue, and black foods a normal part of your nutritional plan.
12. Find ways to rest and recover.

CHAPTER S

Emotional Health

Setting Healthy Boundaries

Check out www.rhondahuff.com for the video lesson, "Chapter S"

Boundaries, an incredible book by Henry Cloud and John Townsend, helped me to see myself as a person who deserved respect from others. I was raised in a typical Christian home where I was always taught to put others before myself. And while I still believe in the basic principle, I have learned that by setting appropriate boundaries, I am able to do that more effectively and from a healthier place within myself.

In the past, I sacrificed my own sanity and priorities to do whatever other people needed me to do. This led to burn-out and a type of mental exhaustion that left me feeling like I wasn't being effective in any area of my life.

Boundaries helped me see that the Biblical idea of putting others first needed some clarification. By putting healthy boundaries around my time, my money, my family, my emotional health, and the way I allowed another human to treat me, I began to heal areas of my life that had been in turmoil for years. One crucial area was my marriage. I believed in "for better or worse" to a fault. I hated divorce and believed God would hate me if I divorced my husband, even though he had been abusive throughout the entire twenty-eight years of our marriage. I read this book during a time when I had left him. I had left many times before only to go back after he promised to get help and change. I would go back with renewed hope only to find that, in two or three months, things were back where they had been. No progress whatsoever. There is a section in "Boundaries" that discusses this type of situation, and the authors make it clear that while reconciliation is the goal, you should not return to a situation until you see genuine and sustained change for an extended time. Unfortunately, in my situation, my husband wasn't willing to do the work or wait. He filed for divorce six months later after offering me an ultimatum: "Would you rather go back to the way things were six months ago or see me with another woman?" My instant reply was, "See you with another woman. I will never go back to the way it was." And that was the end of that.

The book is set up by topic so skip around and read the chapters you need the most. Record areas that need work with one or two action steps to help you set appropriate boundaries around your life. Boundaries are not walls. They are fences, fences that allow good things in and keep bad things out.

Boundary Needed	Action Step 1	Action Step 2

Other observations:

_____

_____

_____

_____

_____

_____

_____

_____

_____

Nutritional Health

Superfoods

When I think of superfoods, I envision food flying in with red capes on, promising to save the day. I believe any whole food is a superfood, bringing essential nutrients to our bodies.

Here is a list of what researchers have found to carry the most nutrients, warranting the term, superfood. Look through the list and circle the foods you are willing to try and then work to get more of them into your nutritional plan.

Vegetables: beets, broccoli, Brussels sprouts, cabbage, carrots, dandelion, kale, mushrooms, onions, spinach, Swiss chard, watercress

Grains: oatmeal, quinoa

Beans and legumes: beans, lentils

Fruits: avocados, blueberries, cherries, coconut, guava, kiwi, raspberries, strawberries

Nuts, seeds, and nut butters: almonds/almond butter, pecans, walnuts

Dairy: butter/ghee, raw organic milk, yogurt/kefir/lassi

Meat, poultry and eggs: eggs

Seafood: sardines, wild Alaskan salmon

Specialty foods: bee pollen/propolis/royal jelly, barley grass/wheatgrass/algae, kimchi, sauerkraut, sea vegetables (seaweed), sprouts

Beverages: fresh vegetable juice, noni juice, pomegranate juice, tea (green, black, white), water

Herbs, spices and condiments: cinnamon, garlic, ginger, oregano, turmeric

Oils: coconut, extra virgin olive, flaxseed, macadamia nut

Physical Health

Sets and Reps

When resistance training, your goals, fitness level, and body type should help guide your program. And everyone should have a program. Without a program you are just guessing. It is helpful to monitor work and progress in order to reach your training goals. Here is a simple guideline to help you progress from where you are now. There are many different ways to do this and there are many different theories around sets and reps.

If you use fitness magazines to design your workout program you may have read that three sets of ten is optimal—for everything—and that's the problem. Let's think about this a minute. Let's say you are doing a four-day split: chest and biceps/back and triceps/shoulders and abs/legs. It may not make sense to do the same set/rep scheme for your small muscle groups as you do the large muscle groups. Anytime you work chest (pushing exercises), you are also working triceps and anytime you work back (pulling exercises) you are also working biceps. So, over the course of the four days, you are doing thirty exercises each for the chest and back and sixty exercises each for the biceps and triceps. Doesn't really make much sense does it?

According to www.t-nation.com it really isn't about the sets anyway. It is about the reps and doing the correct number of reps no matter how many sets it takes. As with everything in the *Healthy Living from A to Z* program, use the information as a starting place, keep good records, and determine how your body responds. Then adjust as needed.

Think about your goal for each body part. And think about symmetry. Then try the following guidelines as you set up your program.

Goal	Rep goal for set 1	Total Reps	Rest between sets
Strength	4-6	25	3 minutes
Hypertrophy (muscle size)	8-12	40	2 minutes
Endurance	15-20	60	less than 1 minute

Ways to progress your workout:

Remember to change it up. Every four to eight weeks you need a new plan. Go back to Chapter E to help guide you so that all movement patterns and muscle actions are trained.

Here's how to mix it up! **Only change one variable at a time.**

Change your Set Type

Circuits: a series of exercises performed one after another, using movements that target all major muscle groups in one continuous cycle with little rest.

Pyramids: start with a moderate load and with each subsequent set, add weight but drop the number of reps performed until you reach muscle fatigue

Supersets: two sequential exercises that target opposing movements such as a chest press and a row (push and pull).

Compound Sets: two (or more) exercises in a row that target the same movement pattern or muscle group.

Complex Sets: a.k.a. post-activation potentiation. Two sequential exercises for the same movement pattern but the first exercise follows the guidelines for strength and after a one to three minute rest, the second exercise follows the guidelines for power. An example would be Barbell Squats followed by Bodyweight Squat Jumps.

Pre-exhaustive Sets: doing exercises to pre-fatigue assistant muscles (synergists) to target the prime mover more exclusively. An example would be to do triceps work before chest work.

Sets for Time: (AMRAP-As Many Reps as Possible) doing as many reps as possible in a pre-determined period of time.

Add Weight
Change reps

If you are working strength, switch it up and work for endurance, etc.

Change tempo

For example…

Concentric (muscle shortening	Pause	Eccentric (muscle lengthening)	Pause
1-2 seconds	1-2 seconds	2-8 seconds	1 second

Add instability

Lower body stability progression: move from a wide base to more of a narrow base. From there you can progress to unilateral movements (one leg), mixed base of support movements (Bulgarian squat), and dynamic movements (adding a hop).

Upper body stability progression: move from seated with back support to seated with no back support to standing, to using an unstable support such as a pushup with one hand on a medicine ball.

Add complexity

Lower body complexity progression: move from bodyweight only movements to weight bearing movements. Then you can add other body movements such as a lunge with an overhead press. You can also begin to change direction with your movements.

Upper body complexity progression: move from bilateral movements to alternating and then to reciprocal and unilateral. You can then progress to adding lower body movements or multiple movements combined.

Remember to track your progress. Your workout should be individualized to your goals, your needs, and your body.

Cognitive Health

Sudoku

I love Sudoku! This New York Times website keeps time. See how you do.

http://www.nytimes.com/crosswords/game/sudoku/easy

http://www.nytimes.com/crosswords/game/sudoku/medium

http://www.nytimes.com/crosswords/game/sudoku/hard

What is your time?

Easy_____

Medium_____

Hard_____

CHAPTER T PREP

1. Begin Chapter T's affirmation.
   I am free to receive happiness in my life.
2. Foam roll daily and before workouts. Do only the corrective exercises that are still difficult for you. After foam rolling, use a dynamic warmup before beginning your workout.
3. Make someone else laugh today.
4. Get your macro- and micro-nutrients each day through wholesome and healthy foods and remember to include prebiotic and probiotic foods! Refer to Chapter G if you need a reminder.
5. Eat your food with a grateful heart. Focus on how many people it took to bring you each meal. From the farmers to the transportation drivers to the grocery store employees to the preparers, to the restaurant staff.
6. Continue to experiment with healthy ways to deal with pain. Don't settle for less than best.
7. Take some time to be quiet every day.
8. Continue to focus on responding not reacting.
9. Find ways to rest and recover.
10. Set appropriate and healthy boundaries and stick to them.

CHAPTER T

Emotional Health

Thought-provoking Questions

Spend some time this week answering the following questions. I ask you to think deeply about them first. We all have our quick "right" answers to life's questions. Don't worry about being "right," be authentic instead.

What stands between you and ultimate happiness?

_____

_____

If you could send a message to the whole world in thirty seconds, what would you say?

_____

_____

_____

If you received enough money to never have to work again, what would you spend your time doing?

_____

_____

If today were your last day on earth, how would you spend it?

_____

_____

_____

If your entire life were a movie, what would be an appropriate title?

_____

_____

_____

How would you describe yourself in five words?

_____

_____

_____

How would you describe your life in five words?

_____

_____

_____

What advice would you give your younger self?

_____

_____

_____

When was the last time you tried something new?

_____

_____

_____

_____

What is the difference between living and existing? Which are you doing?

_____

_____

_____

_____

If you had a friend that spoke to you the way you speak to yourself, how long would you allow that person to be your friend?

_____

_____

_____

_____

What makes you smile?

_____

_____

_____

_____

What can you do today that you couldn't do a year ago?

_____

_____

_____

_____

What do you want most out of life?

_____

_____

_____

_____

What does how you spend your time say about you?

_____

_____

_____

_____

What habits are holding you back from success?

_____

_____

_____

_____

Are you feeding your fears or your dreams?

_____

_____

_____

_____

What is your greatest strength? How do you use it to help others?

_____

_____

_____

_____

Describe your hopes for the future in one sentence.

_____

_____

_____

_____

When did you last push the boundaries of your comfort zone? What was the result?

_____

_____

_____

_____

Deep down, who are you? Describe yourself without using the attributes ascribed to you by others.

_____

_____

_____

Nutritional Health

Taste your Food

Ayurvedic philosophy teaches that all six tastes should be consumed in every meal to enhance satisfaction and to ensure that all major food groups and nutrients are consumed. This week, work to get all six tastes into at least one meal per day.

Taste and Location on Tongue	Predominant Elements and Organs	Basis of Taste	Mind-Body Effect	Food Source
Astringent / Cooling Central region at the back of the tongue	Air and Earth Plasma, Blood, Muscle, Reproductive Tissues	Tannins	• Balances Kapha and Pitta • Excess consumption can aggravate Vata	Apples Avocado Bananas Beans Cabbage Carrots-raw Cauliflower Chicken (light meat) Grape skins Lentils Most raw vegetables Pomegranate Popcorn Tea Venison Wheat pasta
Bitter / Cooling Middle edges of the left and right sides of the tongue and a small band across the middle of the tongue	Air and Ether Plasma, Blood, Fat, Nervous System, Reproductive Tissues	Alkaloids or glycosides	• Balances Kapha and Pitta • Excess consumption can cause gas or indigestion in Vata • Detoxifying to the body	Beets Broccoli Celery Coffee Collards Dandelion greens Dark chocolate Eggplant Green & yellow vegetables Green leafy vegetables Kale Sesame seeds Sprouts

Pungent / Heating Central region of the tongue	Fire and Air Stomach and Heart	Essential Oils	• Balances Kapha • Excess consumption can irritate Pitta and Vata • Promotes sweating • Clears the sinuses	Black pepper Buckwheat Cayenne Chilies Cloves Garlic Ginger Leeks Mustard Mustard greens Onions Peppers Radishes Salsa Spelt Spinach—raw Turnips
Salty / Heating Rear edges of the tongue	Water and Fire Kidneys	Mineral Salts	• Balances Vata • Excess consumption may aggravate Kapha and Pitta • Enhances appetite • Makes other tastes more yummy	Cottage cheese Fish Salt Salted meats Seaweed Tamari
Sour / Heating Front edges of the tongue, along the tapered curve	Earth and Fire Lungs	Organic acids: ascorbic acid, citric acid, acetic acid	• Balances Vata • Excess consumption can aggravate Kapha and Pitta • Stimulates the appetite • Aids digestion	Alcohol Butter Cheese Citrus fruits Pickled foods Raisins Salad dressing Sour cream Tomatoes Yogurt

Sweet / Cooling Tip of the tongue	Earth and Water Thyroid and Upper Lungs	Carbohy-drates, Protein, Fat	• Balances Vata and Pitta • Excess consumption aggravates Kapha • Soothing effect on the body • Satisfying • Builds body mass	Bread Chicken Dairy Fish Grains, pasta Honey Meat Molasses Rice Starch Sugar Vegetables

Physical Health

Total Body Workouts

Check out www.rhondahuff.com for the video lesson, "Chapter T"

My favorite style of training is Total Body Training. Training every muscle in every plane of motion with every joint movement each time you train. It cuts down on how many times you need to train in a week and keeps the body functioning properly through full ranges of motion.

Look back at Chapter I. This is the foundation of a Total Body Workout. Now let's take it to another level. For each workout, make sure you have each of the following elements:

Horizontal PUSH (ex. Push up, Chest Press, Skullcrushers)
Horizontal PULL (ex. Rows of any kind)
Vertical PUSH (ex. Overhead Press, Push Press)
Vertical PULL (ex. Lat Pulldown, Pullups, Bicep Curls)
KNEE Dominant (ex. Squats, Lunges)
HIP Dominant (ex. Deadlift, Glute bridges)
Core
Metabolic
Shoulders, Chest, and Triceps are PUSHERS.
Back and Biceps are PULLERS.

I also use a lot of complex movements that train multiple body parts at once.

Below is an example of a typical training program. I use three circuits of three exercises that are rotated three times. I kept this one simple without a lot of complexity. That should tell you from last week's lesson that this person hasn't been training that long as we have not added much instability or complexity. Using what you have learned thus far, see what else you can determine about this person's goals.

SMR = Self Myofascial Release, a.k.a. foam rolling
KB = Kettebell
BW = Bodyweight
DB = Dumbbell
RDL = Romanian Deadlift

Sets / Reps	Weight	Exercise	Plane/Movement
		SMR	
		Dynamic Warm-up	
		Corrective Work	
3/15	12kg KB	Goblet Squats	Sagittal/Knee Dom
3/8	50 Cable	Lat Pulldowns	Frontal/Vert Pull
3/:30	BW	Inclined Mountain Climbers with External Hip Rotation	Transverse/Metabolic
3/10 each	TRX	Lateral Lunges	Frontal/Knee Dom
3/12	20 DB	Bench Press	Transverse/Hor Push
3/:30	BW	Plank with Renegade Rows	Sagittal/Core/Hor Pull
3/15	24kg KB	RDL	Sagittal/Hip Dom
3/8	12 DB	Overhead Press	Transverse/Vert Push
3/:30	6kg ViPR	Lateral Shuffles	Frontal/Metabolic
		Stretch	

Cognitive Health

Teasers

Check off each task once it is successfully completed. (www.sharpbrains.com is one of many websites with fun brainteasers. See their website for more!)

- Say the days of the week backwards, then in alphabetical order.
- Say the months of the year in alphabetical order.
- Say the months of the year in reverse alphabetical order.
- Using your mind only, find the sum of your date of birth (mm/dd/yyyy).
- Name two objects for every letter in your first name. Work up to five objects, trying to use different items each time.
- Look around wherever you are and, within two minutes, try to find five red things that will fit in your pockets, and five blue objects that are too big to fit.
- Count the number of fs in this sentence, "Finished files are the result of years of scientific study combined with the experience of years."
- A blind beggar had a brother who died. What relation was the blind beggar to the brother who died? "Brother" is not the answer.
- Find a third word that is connected or associated with both of these two words.
  1. LOCK—PIANO
  2. SHIP—CARD
  3. TREE—CAR
  4. SCHOOL—EYE
  5. PILLOW—COURT
  6. RIVER—MONEY
  7. BED—PAPER
  8. ARMY—WATER
  9. TENNIS—NOISE
  10. EGYPTIAN—MOTHER
  11. SMOKER—PLUMBER
- Of one hundred people at a recent party, ninety spoke Spanish, eighty spoke Italian, and seventy-five spoke Mandarin. At least how many spoke all three languages?

All teasers taken from www.sharpbrains.com

Solutions:

- Sunday, Saturday, Friday, Thursday, Wednesday, Tuesday, Monday. Friday, Monday, Saturday, Sunday, Thursday, Tuesday, Wednesday.
- April, August, December, February, January, July, June, March, May, November, October, September
- September, October, November, May, March, June, July, January, February, December, August, April
- Did you add individual numbers or the sum of each section? For example I am 11/16/1964 so the sum of my digits is 29 but the sum of the 3 sections is 1991.
- Robin/rotator cuff, hat/hairspray, onion/oncologist, nest/nightshades, dinner/diamond, apple/anteater. ?anteater?
- Pencil, shoestring, bottle top, paper, tissue paper. Sandal, water bottle, book, CD box, robe
- 6
- The blind beggar was the sister of her brother, who died.
  1. LOCK—PIANO > Key
  2. SHIP—CARD > Deck
  3. TREE—CAR > Trunk
  4. SCHOOL—EYE > Pupil (Exam and Private are also possible)
  5. PILLOW—COURT > Case
  6. RIVER—MONEY > Bank (Flow is also possible)
  7. BED—PAPER > Sheet
  8. ARMY—WATER > Tank
  9. TENNIS—NOISE > Racket
  10. EGYPTIAN—MOTHER > Mummy
  11. SMOKER—PLUMBER > Pipe
- 45: Ten could not speak Spanish, twenty could not speak Italian, and twenty-five could not speak Mandarin. So, there could have been ten people who spoke none of those languages. However, that would maximize the number of people who could speak all three, and the problem asks at least how many speak all three. Therefore, we must assume that these ten, twenty, and twenty-five people are all separate people. Having identified fifty-five each of whom is missing one language, the remaining forty-five speak all three.

All teasers taken from www.sharpbrains.com

CHAPTER U PREP

1. Begin Chapter U's affirmation.
   I am taking control of my health.
2. Foam roll daily and before workouts. Do only the corrective exercises that are still difficult for you. After foam rolling, use a dynamic warmup before beginning your workout.
3. Take a few moments to watch something funny. I love to watch children and animals. Just pure entertainment. Try to belly-laugh like a child. Go ahead, no one can see you!
4. Get your macro- and micro-nutrients each day through wholesome and healthy foods.
5. Take some time to be quiet every day. Pray, meditate, dream. What do you want your future to look like? Dream about that.
6. Are you able to respond with respect? Keep working on that.
7. Find ways to rest and recover.
8. Set appropriate and healthy boundaries and stick to them.
9. Continue to experiment with all six tastes. Try something new!
10. Try some total body workouts this week. Try programming a smart workout following this outline:
    a. SMR (Self-Myofascial Release—Foam Rolling) times five minutes
    b. Warm-up all joints and muscles times five minutes

c. Circuit 1 times three sets (roughly ten minutes)
  i. Lower Body Exercise
  ii. Upper Body Exercise
  iii. Metabolic or Core Exercise
d. Circuit 2 times three sets (roughly ten minutes)
  i. Lower Body Exercise
  ii. Upper Body Exercise
  iii. Metabolic or Core Exercise
e. Circuit 3 times three sets (roughly ten minutes)
  i. Lower Body Exercise
  ii. Upper Body Exercise
  iii. Metabolic or Core Exercise
f. Cool down / Stretch times five to ten minutes

CHAPTER U

Emotional Health

Unmasked

Check out www.rhondahuff.com for the video lesson, "Chapter U"

Over the last twenty chapters, we have worked on becoming authentic, bold, and centered and we have discussed how this begins in the mind and directly affects our nutritional, physical, and cognitive health practices.

If you have done the emotional work and are harboring no more masks that cover your true self, then this is a time of celebration and reflection for you! Congratulations on your hard work and becoming unmasked.

If you feel that you haven't yet arrived at this accomplishment, then I invite you to take some time to remove any mask that still covers your true self. Here is a guideline to help you out.

The mask I can't take off is:

_____

_____

_____

The reason I haven't taken off this mask is:

_____

_____

_____

This reason exists because of (This may be an incident or a person—be as specific as possible and if you can't remember, use the hypnosis video in Chapter H to allow your subconscious to bring it to mind):

_____

_____

_____

What would happen if I removed this mask?

_____

_____

_____

How would my life be different without this mask?

_____

_____

_____

How would the removal of this mask affect those around me?

_____

_____

_____

What may be the long-term consequences of continuing to wear this mask?

_____

_____

_____

Today I am WILLING / UNWILLING to remove this mask and live as my authentic self.

If you are unwilling, it's OK. Return to this exercise another time.

If you are willing, map out a plan, including a support system that can help you remain in a place of authenticity. For me, this support system includes my closest friends who love me unconditionally and know that I tend to be extremely hard on myself and put up an I-can-handle-everything-all-by-myself front. They don't hesitate to jerk that mask right off my face and force me to open up and allow others to help me when needed. In the beginning, this felt very much like failure and a "parental" reprimand. Now it is welcomed and appreciated. And I am happy to report that it isn't as necessary as before because I have learned to reach out BEFORE the moment of crisis hits. And if you really think about it, isn't this one of the purposes of friends and family? To love unconditionally, to carry one another's' burdens, and to "sharpen one another's iron (Proverbs 27:17)?" The key may be to find the ones who truly do love you unconditionally. It is only in love that anything else can be done with a pure heart and motive. If you don't have those people in your life, begin to pray for God to send that type of person to you. It makes life much more fun and burdens much more bearable.

The friend(s) or family member that I know will help me remove this mask once and for all is:

I will contact this person on this date:

Here is how I will explain what I am doing and how he/she can help me:

Nutritional Health

Understanding Food Labels

Food labeling regulations fall primarily under the jurisdiction of two federal agencies: the Food and Drug Administration (FDA) and the United States Department of Agriculture (USDA). They define two categories of claims: nutrient content claims and health claims. Nutrient content claims are statements about the level of a nutrient in a food. Health claims link the nutrient profile of a food to a health or disease condition.

Labels must contain:

Product Identity Statement
    Food form and type, i.e. *diced tomatoes*
Manufacturer's Name and Address
    Net Quantity of Contents
Weight, measure, or counts
    List of Ingredients
In descending order of predominance
    Ingredients in amounts less than 2 percent of the product do not have to be listed
Nutrition Facts Statement
    Required Nutrients: fourteen must be listed
    Percent Daily Value: based on a 2,000-calorie-per-day diet
    Serving Size: the amount customarily eaten at one time

So, I just want to point out a few things.

1. Customarily eaten at one time: By whom? How old is this person? How big is this person? A 35-pound kid versus a 100-pound teenager versus a 200-pound man should not customarily be eating the same amount at one time.

2. Based on a 2,000-calorie-per-day diet: Once again, how do you know if you are supposed to be eating 2,000 calories? Typically, this is too much for a grown female and not enough for a grown male. It is also too much for kids and not enough for athletes.

3. The List of Ingredients is by far THE MOST IMPORTANT part of the label. Don't get too caught up in how many calories or fat or sugar. If the first few ingredients are sugar (or a sugar substance), a saturated or trans fat, or salt in any form, you should leave it on the shelf. Remember the F in FOOD© is for

free of anti-nutrients. If you can't pronounce it or don't know what it is, leave it on the shelf.

I am sure you have learned by now that in most cases, if the food needs a label, it may not be a great source of nutrition. Whole foods don't need labels. You know what's in an apple or lettuce or grass-fed beef. No labels needed.

Make a concerted effort to eat foods that don't require nutrition facts labels. And if you are eating out, you won't know if the pineapple you are eating came out of a can or was cut fresh. You can certainly ask. You can also choose to eat at home.

Physical Health

Unilateral Training

NOTE: Unilateral training is a PROGRESSION. Never jump right into unilateral training without proper planning and programming.

Unilateral training is simply training limbs individually instead of together. If you do lunges or one-arm rows, you are training unilaterally. I love unilateral training for a few reasons:

1. It is more functional. Other than squatting to sit, nearly everything we do in life requires unilateral movement: walking, eating, climbing stairs, opening doors, brushing teeth, stirring a pot of soup, reaching for something high on a shelf, writing, pulling a wagon, kicking a soccer ball, carrying a bag of groceries, running, etc.

2. Thanks to number one, above, we are often left with imbalances between our dominant and nondominant side. Therefore, unilateral training allows us to correct those imbalances. Here are two ways to do that:

   a. Do an exercise with the nondominant side to failure. Then only train the dominant side to that number until the nondominant side can do more. For example, if you can lift a fifteen-pound dumbbell ten times with your left arm and only seven times with your right arm, do sets of seven reps on both arms and increase together.

   b. Do two sets for the nondominant side for every set on the dominant side. Using the same example above, lift the dumbbell seven times on the right, ten times on the left, and another seven (or whatever you can get) on the right.

3. Reduces bilateral deficit. Believe it or not, the whole is not usually equal to the sum of its parts where muscular strength is concerned. In most cases you can train unilaterally **heavier** than you can bilaterally!

4. Unilateral training trains core stability and works on balance much more than bilateral training. In a single arm chest press, for example, it is much harder to control the core and maintain balance than in a double arm chest press.

5. It is a great PROGRESSION. Remember the chapter on sets and reps. Unilateral movement is number four on the upper body complexity progression list (bilateral, alternating, reciprocating, unilateral). It is number three on lower body stability progression list (wide base, narrow base, stable unilateral base). So be smart with your programming. Don't jump into unilateral training without going through the appropriate progressions first.

Cognitive Health

Unraveling Cognitive Decline...Prevention is KEY
According to the Alzheimer's Association, there are four lifestyle habits that can reduce your risk of cognitive decline:

1. Physical health and exercise: break a sweat, get your heart rate up to increase blood circulation to your body and brain

2. Diet and nutrition: follow the FOOD© principle

3. Cognitive activity: although there is little evidence that puzzles, crosswords, etc. can actually reverse cognitive decline, it has been shown that such activities may help ward off cognitive decline. It is also suggested that timed activities where you are working to get faster at the decision-making portion of those activities stimulates brain cells. So, when doing those activities, set a timer and beat the clock! Also, anytime you learn something new, the brain changes and neuronal connections become stronger and dendrites become fatter with myelin, which reduces interference allowing signals to travel faster. Remember, learning is ongoing. You must practice what you are learning. The information must make its way into long-term memory. And also remember that *practice makes permanent, only **perfect** practice makes perfect.*

4. Social engagement: make friends, establish positive and healthy connections and relationships

The *Healthy Living from A to Z* program is designed to help with the first three areas. While there is an opportunity for social engagement, the best social engagement is face-to-face interaction.

Take some time this week to review past chapters that may need a little boost. And then talk to people about what you are learning—face-to-face!

If you can teach it, you understand it!

CHAPTER V PREP

1. Begin Chapter V's affirmation. (Do you still use your taped-off mirror? I hope so!)
   My heart and lungs are getting healthier every single day.
2. Foam roll daily and before workouts. Do only the corrective exercises that are still difficult for you. After foam rolling, use a dynamic warmup before beginning your workout.
3. Continue to take some time to be quiet every day.
4. Look back on how differently people respond to you when you respond instead of react. Can you see, feel, and hear a difference? Write down your thoughts:

   _____
   _____
   _____
   _____

5. What have become your favorite ways to rest and recover?

   _____
   _____
   _____
   _____

6. How are you doing with setting appropriate boundaries?
7. Continue to experiment with all six tastes. Share a new recipe with a friend.

8. What mask are you wearing right now? How easily can it be removed?

9. Are you getting better at reading food labels? This is so important!

10. Create a cognitive decline prevention plan. Remember to include all the foundational elements: Exercise, nutrition, cognitive activity, social engagement. Write down your plan:

_____

_____

_____

_____

CHAPTER V

Emotional Health

Vocalizing the Song Within

> *I don't sing because I'm happy; I'm happy because I sing.*
> —**William James**, Father of American Psychology

Research shows that singing creates an internal environment that combines a calming of the nerves and a lifting of the spirit. The calming effect comes from the lowering of the stress hormone, cortisol, while the lifting comes from the release of endorphins and oxytocin, both of which creates feelings of pleasure and the alleviation of anxiety, depression, and loneliness. The oxytocin release is elevated even more when singing with a group, creating a sense of trust and bonding. Another area of research suggests that when singing in a group, the entire groups' heart rates sync up, creating an environment very similar to guided group meditation.

Even if it's in the shower alone, sing! Find the song within and allow it to strengthen your health and elevate your happiness.

Nutritional Health

Vitamins

Essential vitamins are those that you must obtain from outside sources in order for the body to work properly. These sources are usually food, but in the case of Vitamin D, it is primarily sunlight. The thirteen essential vitamins are:

A, D, E, K, C, B1, B2, B3, B5, B6, B7, B9, B12

- Help promote and regulate various chemical reactions and bodily processes
- Participate in releasing energy from food

Mild vitamin deficiencies are common in senior adults and in people who take certain prescription medications.

Vitamin	RDA	Why it is important	Sources
Vitamin B1 Thiamine	1.4 mg	Maintenance of cellular and organ functions. Deficiency can lead to a breakdown of the nervous and circulatory systems and in rare cases, the development of beriberi and/or Wernicke-Korsakoff syndrome. Over-consumption is unknown and studies show that amounts taken well in excess of the DV can actually enhance brain functioning.	yeast extract spread (marmite), sesame seeds, tahini, sunflower seeds, dried coriander, poppy seeds, sage paprika, mustard seed, rosemary, thyme, pork chops, pine nuts, pistachios, macadamia nuts, pecans, pompano, tuna

| Vitamin B2 Riboflavin | 1.7 mg | Maintenance of proper energy metabolism and many cellular processes. Deficiency can lead to cracking and reddening of the lips, inflammation of the mouth, mouth ulcers, sore throat, and possibly an iron deficiency or anemia. Overdose is rare since it is a water-soluble vitamin that is well regulated by the body and usually only occurs during vitamin B2 injections. | yeast extract spread (marmite), liver, dried ancho chilies, paprika coriander, spearmint, parsley, chili powder, almonds, wheat bran, mackerel, salmon, trout, sesame seeds |

| Vitamin B3 Niacin | 20 mg | Needed for the processing of fat in the body, lowering cholesterol and regulating blood sugar levels.

Deficiency, along with a deficiency of tryptophan causes pellagra. Symptoms include aggression, dermatitis, insomnia, weakness, mental confusion, and diarrhea. In advanced cases, pellagra may lead to dementia and death.

Even a slight deficiency of niacin can lead to irritability, poor concentration, anxiety, fatigue, restlessness, apathy, and depression.

It is well regulated by the body and overdosing only occurs when niacin is taken in the form of supplements. An overdose of niacin is seen in the form of skin rashes, dry skin, and digestive problems.

A long-term overdose can lead to liver damage, elevated blood sugar levels and type II diabetes, as well as increased risk of birth defects. | yeast extract spread (marmite), rice and wheat bran, anchovies, tuna, swordfish, liver, paprika, peanuts, veal, chicken (light meat), bacon, sun-dried tomatoes |

Vitamin B5 Pantothenic Acid	10 mg	Maintenance of cellular processes and fat metabolism. Deficiency is rare. However, when it does occur it is usually seen in the form of irritability, fatigue, apathy, numbness, paresthesia, and muscle cramps. It can also lead to increased sensitivity to insulin, or hypoglycemia.	liver, rice and wheat bran, sunflower seeds, mushrooms, caviar, cheese, sun-dried tomatoes, fish, avocados
Vitamin B6 Pyridoxine	2 mg	Maintenance of red blood cell metabolism, the nervous system, the immune system, and many other bodily functions. Over time, a deficiency in vitamin B-6 can lead to skin inflammation (dermatitis) depression, confusion, convulsions, and even anemia. Recent studies also suggest that a diet low in vitamin B6 increases risk of heart attack. Conversely, too much vitamin B6 from supplements can lead to nerve damage in the arms and legs.	rice and wheat bran, dried chili powder, paprika, garlic powder, tarragon, ground sage, spearmint, basil, chives, savory, turmeric, bay leaves, rosemary, dill, onion powder, oregano, and marjoram , pistachios, garlic, liver, tuna, salmon, cod, tahini, sunflower seeds, pork loin, sorghum, molasses, hazelnuts

Vitamin B7 (aka Vitamin H—from the German words for "hair" and "skin", *Haar und Haut*) Biotin	Scientists say intestinal bacteria most likely produce vitamin B7 in quantities beyond our daily requirements. Hence, government health departments in most countries do not recommend daily intake amounts.	Metabolism of proteins, fats and carbohydrates, the processing of glucose, transference of CO2, maintenance of healthy nails, skin and hair. (However, it cannot be absorbed through hair or skin.) Vitamin B7 deficiency is extremely rare.	green peas, broccoli, cabbage, cauliflower, sweet potatoes, spinach, bananas, avocados, strawberries, raspberries, watermelon, grapefruit, oats, soybeans, wheatgerm, lentils, split peas, bran, unpolished brown rice almonds, pecans, peanuts walnuts, Brewer's yeast, egg yolks, liver
Vitamin B9 Folate (when occurring naturally in foods) Folic Acid (is the synthetic form of folate – choose folate instead)	400 mcg	DNA synthesis and repair, cell division, and cell growth. A deficiency of folate can lead to anemia in adults, and slower development in children. For pregnant women, folate is especially important for proper fetal development. Overdose is rare in natural food sources and only occurs from supplements.	yeast extract, dried spearmint, basil, rosemary, chervil, coriander, marjoram, thyme, bay leaf, parsley, liver, sunflower seeds, spinach, turnip greens, collards, pea sprouts, garbanzo beans, mung beans, pinto beans, asparagus, peanuts

| Vitamin B12 Cobalamin | RDA is based on age: Under 12 months: 0.4—0.5 mcg Ages 1 to 3: 0.9 mcg Ages 4 to 8: 1.2mcg Ages 9 to 13: 1.8mcg Over 14 years: 2.4mcg Pregnant women: 2.6mcg Breastfeeding women: 2.8mcg | B12 is the largest and most complex vitamin currently known to man. Keeps the body's nerve and blood cells healthy, helps make DNA, helps prevent megaloblastic anemia A slight deficiency of vitamin B-12 can lead to anemia, fatigue, mania, and depression, while a long-term deficiency can cause permanent damage to the brain and central nervous system. Vitamin B12 can only be manufactured by bacteria and can only be found naturally in animal products, however, synthetic forms are widely available and added to many foods. Vitamin B12 can be consumed in large doses because excess is excreted by the body or stored in the liver for use when supplies are scarce. Stores of B12 can last for up to a year. | clams, oysters, mussels, liver, caviar, octopus, fish, crab, lobster, lamb, beef, cheese, eggs *Vegetarians and people not eating these foods, may need to supplement* |

Vitamin C Ascorbic Acid	60 mg	Development and maintenance of scar tissue, blood vessels, and cartilage. Vitamin C is also necessary for creating ATP, dopamine, peptide hormones, and tyrosine. As a powerful antioxidant, vitamin C helps lessen oxidative stress to the body and is thought to lower cancer risk. Deficiency can cause fatigue, mood changes, weight loss, joint and muscle aches, bruising, dry hair and skin, infections, and periodontal disease (in its most severe case, scurvy).	red and green hot chili peppers, guavas, bell peppers, thyme, parsley, kale, mustard greens, garden cress, broccoli, cauliflower, Brussels sprouts, kiwi, papaya, oranges, clementine, strawberries
Vitamin A Retinol	5000 IU	Maintains healthy vision, gene transcription, immune function, and great skin health. A deficiency in vitamin A can lead to blindness and increased viral infections. However, deficiency is only considered a problem in developing countries where it is a leading cause of blindness in children. Over consumption of vitamin A can lead to jaundice, nausea, loss of appetite, irritability, vomiting, and hair loss.	eggs, butter, fish, liver, carrots, spinach, sweet potatoes, paprika, red pepper, cayenne pepper, chili powder, dark leafy greens, butternut squash, red and green leaf lettuce, dried apricots

| Vitamin D Calciferol | The current U.S. DV for vitamin D is 600 IU (international units) and the toxicity threshold for vitamin D is thought to be 10,000 to 40,000 IU/day.2 Vitamin D is oil soluble, which means you need to eat fat to absorb it. | Assists the absorption of calcium, bone development, cell growth, neuromuscular functioning, immune functioning, and alleviation of inflammation. Inadequate levels of vitamin D can lead to a weakened immune system, increased cancer risk, poor hair growth, and osteomalacia, a condition of weakened muscles and bones. A severe deficiency can lead to rickets, a disease in which bones fail to properly develop. Excess vitamin D can cause the body to absorb too much calcium, leading to increased risk of heart attack and kidney stones. | cod liver oil, fish, oysters, caviar, mushrooms, egg yolks. The skin makes vitamin D when exposed to sunlight. As little as five to thirty minutes without sunscreen a few times a week may be enough for most people. |

| Vitamin E Tocopherols and Tocotrienols | 20 mg | Vitamin E is a group of eight fat-soluble vitamins that help prevent oxidative stress to the body.

Adequate amounts of vitamin E can help protect against heart disease, cancer, and age-related eye damage (macular degeneration).

An overdose from supplements can lead to excessive bleeding, or hemorrhaging.

Vitamin E deficiencies are rare but can be seen in people with an inability to absorb dietary fats and in premature infants. | sunflower seeds, paprika, red chili powder, almonds, pine nuts, peanuts, basil, oregano, dried apricots, pickled green olives, cooked spinach, cooed taro root, avocado |

Vitamin K Phytona-dione	80 mcg	Required for protein modification and blood clotting. Recent studies suggest that vitamin K may play a role in treating osteoporosis and Alzheimer's, and that consuming increased levels of vitamin K can help protect against cancer and heart disease. Risk alert: medications to prevent blood clots, like Warfarin or Coumadin, cannot be combined with vitamin K and even foods high in vitamin K should be cleared with your doctor. Vitamin K deficiency is rare in adults. However, people with liver disease, pancreatic disease, celiac disease, bulimia, inflammatory bowel disease, people on strict diets, people with malabsorption, or people who have had abdominal surgeries are at a higher risk. A deficiency will yield bleeding disorders such as nose bleeds, heavy menstrual bleeding, bleeding gums, broken blood vessels, easy bruising, and blood in the urine.	dried basil, sage, thyme, dark leafy greens, scallions, broccoli, asparagus, chili powder, curry, paprika, cayenne, cabbage, pickled cucumber, prunes

Physical Health

VO₂ Max (Volume of Oxygen)

VO_2 max is a numerical measurement of your body's ability to consume oxygen. It is measured in milliliters per kilograms of body weight per minute (ml/kg/min). It is a simple way to check your cardiovascular fitness level.

As exercise effort increases, the amount of oxygen you consume to produce energy (and the rate at which you exhale carbon dioxide) increases. However, there is a maximum level of oxygen consumption, beyond which increases in exercise intensity don't lead to further increases in oxygen consumption. This level of oxygen consumption is called the VO2 max.

The higher the number the better as it means that your body can take in more oxygen and deliver it to your muscles, producing more energy thus producing more work.

For truly accurate results, you would need to go to a clinic with the proper testing tools. But to get a general idea and a baseline with which to work toward improvement, follow the protocol below.

1. Foam roll and warmup
2. Set a treadmill to an incline of one
3. Run and/or walk for twelve minutes
4. Record distance
5. Cool down before stopping
6. Use this formula to determine VO_2 Max
   (35.97 x *distance covered*) – 11.29
   My VO_2 Max is_____
7. Refer to the Norms chart on the page

Non-Athletes Norms		
Age	Male	Female
10-19	47-56	38-46
20-29	43-52	33-42
30-39	39-48	30-38
40-49	36-44	26-35
50-59	34-41	24-33
60-69	31-38	22-30
70-79	28-35	20-27

If your number falls below the norms for your age and sex, set a goal to improve it.

High Intensity Interval Training (HIIT) is one of the best ways to improve your VO_2 Max. This can be as little as twelve minutes per week and can be spread out over three days at four minutes of HIIT each day. Here is a basic guideline for programming a HIIT workout:

- Choose your cardio equipment.
- Warm up for three minutes.
- Exercise as hard and fast as you can for thirty seconds. You should be gasping for breath and feel like you couldn't possibly go on another few seconds.
- Recover for ninety seconds, **still moving** (remember to NEVER come to a stop after exercising), but at slower pace and decreased resistance.
- Repeat the high-intensity exercise and recovery.
- Progress by increasing work or decreasing recovery. Remember to change one variable at a time.
- Cool down for a few minutes afterward by cutting down your intensity by 50 to 80 percent.
- Retest in six weeks.

Cognitive Health

Vibrations

Check out www.rhondahuff.com for the video lesson, "Chapter V"

Brain Wave Vibrations is a form of meditation that has been around for thousands of years. The practice stimulates the brain stem, calms higher frequency brain wave activity, and stimulates the flow of chi (energy), bringing the body and brain back into balance.

Brain Wave Vibration works to bring up water energy and bring down fire energy. Therefore, it is very helpful for balancing the fire Dosha, Pitta. It is also extremely beneficial if you feel yourself getting frustrated or angry, as it will cool the brain.

Brain Wave Vibration has three distinct elements:

1. Deliberately create vibrations within the body. Begin slowly and gently shaking the head "no" moving at the atlas/axis (C1/C2—where the skull meets the spine)
2. Allow the body to ride the rhythm. Move the body parts that want to move
3. Follow the flow of chi. You can add a gentle tapping to the Danjun area (3 inches below the belly button) to enhance digestion and further quiet the mind.

CHAPTER W PREP

1. Begin Chapter W's affirmation.
   I have the power to turn my weaknesses into strengths.
2. Foam roll daily and before workouts. Do only the corrective exercises that are still difficult for you. After foam rolling, use a dynamic warmup before beginning your workout.
3. Continue to focus on responding not reacting.
4. Find ways to rest and recover.
5. Set appropriate and healthy boundaries and stick to them.
6. Continue to experiment with all six tastes.
7. Remain unmasked.
8. Work on your cognitive decline prevention plan.
9. Take some time today to sing at the top of your lungs!
10. Take only the vitamins you know your body needs.
11. Use Brain Wave Vibration when you feel you need a time-out.
12. Take some time to glance back over all of your notes thus far in the program. What have you learned? How have you applied what you are learning to your own life? Have you become more authentic, bold, and centered in your health endeavors?

CHAPTER W

Emotional Health

Weaknesses are Strengths Misused

Check out www.rhondahuff.com for the video lesson, "Chapter W"

Have you ever stopped to consider that the bully on the playground may have amazing leadership skills but has never been taught how to properly lead? Or that the child who cries all the time may be full of empathy and compassion and hasn't developed the necessary skills to handle those emotions?

About 20 years ago, I heard a teacher make a remarkable statement that changed how I looked at others and myself. She simply said, "Every weakness is a strength misused. Find the strength and guide it in the right direction."

How would things be different if all of us would look at our own character traits this way? If every time we spotted a weakness we could find the potential strength and work to gain the wisdom and skills necessary to execute that strength properly, it would replace the negative without leaving a void.

This week take some time to look at your perceived weaknesses. If you think you don't have any, ask your spouse or someone close to you. Then work to discover the potential strength behind that weakness and devise one action step to turn the weakness into a strength.

Perceived Weakness	Potential Strength	Action Step

Nutritional Health

Water

The human body is 60 percent to 75 percent water. The body loses water through respiration, perspiration, urination, and defecation.

Most people say they don't drink enough water. But how much is enough? Where did the eight glasses a day come from and is it accurate? Is it true that by the time we are thirsty, it is too late because we are already dehydrated? Does alcohol and caffeinated drinks count against us? And can we drink too much water?

First let's cover the likely origination of the eight-glasses-a-day rule. In 1945, the Food and Nutrition Board of the National Research Council declared "a suitable allowance of water for adults is 2.5 liters daily in most instances. An ordinary standard is 1 milliliter for each calorie of food. Most of this quantity is contained in prepared foods." Most people who cite this study neglect to cite the last sentence nor relate it to calories per food item.

How much is enough? It depends on your size, health, activity level, and where you live. The larger you are, the more you need. The less healthy you are, the more you need. The more active you are, the more you need. The hotter the climate in which you live, the more you need.

The *Clinical Journal of Sport Medicine* suggests, "Using the innate thirst mechanism to guide fluid consumption is a strategy that should limit drinking in excess and developing hyponatremia while providing sufficient fluid to prevent excessive dehydration." It has been disproven time and time again that once we feel thirst it is too late. Drink when you feel thirsty.

Past recommendations for alcohol and caffeinated drinks suggest a 2:1 ratio of water to alcohol or caffeinated drinks. While water is the healthiest choice, research indicates that the liquid needs for the body encompasses all liquids and also foods that have a high water-content, such as soups, fruits, and vegetables. If your nutrition plan consists of mostly dry (such as bread and meat) or processed foods, you will need to add more fluids during the day. One specific study from the University of Bath, UK, showed no difference in hydration levels when comparing moderate coffee drinkers (four cups per day) to water drinkers.

When working out, too much water can be as harmful as too little. The condition is known as Exercise-Associated Hyponatremia (EAH), in which the kidneys become overwhelmed by the large quantity of liquid it is being forced to process. The blood's naturally occurring sodium levels can't keep up with the amount of water, leading to swelling in the cells and in severe cases, death. Symptoms include lightheadedness, dizziness, nausea, puffiness, and weight gain during a physical activity. In severe cases, vomiting, headaches, confusion, agitation, delirium, seizures, and comas may occur, which can be life-threatening.

The bottom line is to drink when you are thirsty. Here are some basic guidelines that should be used as such: a place to start. Each individual needs to determine what fluid intake is optimal for him or her.

Remember that these guidelines are for TOTAL fluid intake per day. For children, pediatricians recommend that most of the amount be from water and the rest from proper foods. And remember that excessive exercise and severely hot climates may indicate a need for increased hydration.

Age	Amount for boys	Amount for girls
1-3	4 cups	4 cups
4-8	5 cups	5 cups
9-13	8 cups	7 cups
14+	½ your body weight in ounces	½ your body weight in ounces

Physical Health

Weight Training

Weight training can be traced back to ancient Greece where the wrestler, Milo of Croton, carried a calf on his back until it was fully grown. In its simplest form, weight training is defined as "physical training that involves lifting weights." It is used specifically for developing the strength and size of skeletal muscles by utilizing the force of gravity in the form of weighted bars, dumbbells, specialized equipment, and your own body weight in order to oppose the force generated by muscle through concentric or eccentric contractions.

When weight training, proper form and execution is critical in order to get the desired results in a safe way. See Chapter Q for a review of common training errors and how to correct them and also Chapter R for a review of reps and sets.

It is a myth that women shouldn't or can't lift heavy and that it will make them big like men. Unless there are anabolic aids or an extremely muscular genetic body type, a woman will not gain enough size to "look like a man." Women, lifting heavy (usually in the five-rep to eight-rep range) is a great way to train for several reasons. The joints sustain less wear and tear. It builds tremendous confidence. It more effectively burns fat due to EPOC (Excess Post-exercise Oxygen Consumption). It increases energy. It adds curve and tone to the body. It promotes better sleep. It improves bone density and strength, staving off osteoporosis. It tremendously helps with lowering stress levels.

Take a look at your training program. Are you using added weight to reach your goals? If you are, great! Make sure the program is balanced and throw some *heavy* weight training in there. If you aren't, give it a try! Remember quality over quantity (Chapter Q)!

Cognitive Health

Wrinkles

Have you ever heard that every time you learn something new, your brain gets a new wrinkle? Well, turns out that's not true. By the time a fetus is forty weeks old, it has all the wrinkles it will ever have as long as the brain stays healthy. Throughout the first forty weeks of fetal development, neurons grow and migrate to different areas of the brain, creating sulci (the crevices) and gyri (the ridges).

While the brain does change when we learn something new, it does not result in the creation of more wrinkles but it does enhance brain plasticity, also called neuroplasticity. It is a common term used by neuroscientists, referring to the brain's ability to change at any age—for better or worse.

If this is the first time you learned about the "wrinkles" myth, bravo! You just had an exercise in brain plasticity.

CHAPTER X PREP

1. Begin Chapter X's affirmation.
   I choose to live my life, not a Xerox copy of someone else's.
2. Foam roll daily and before workouts. Do only the corrective exercises that are still difficult for you. After foam rolling, use a dynamic warmup before beginning your workout.
3. How are you doing with setting boundaries? If you are struggling, I recommend you actually purchase and read Drs. Cloud and Townsend's book. It can be life changing.
4. Have you mastered getting those 6 tastes into your daily meals?
5. Remain unmasked.
6. Take only the vitamins you know your body needs.
7. Use Brain Wave Vibration when you feel you need a time-out.
8. Find the strengths behind your weaknesses and make a plan to turn them into usable strengths that will bless others.

CHAPTER X

Emotional Health

Xeroxing Life

Check out www.rhondahuff.com for the video lesson, "Chapter X"

I love being able to keep up with my friends from all over the world through the use of social media. However, I also know how tempting it is to covet someone else's life, or at least the life I think they have. Has this ever happened to you?

We live vicariously through other people by following their every post, imagining how much fun it would be to be in their shoes, on their vacations, in their jobs. And we try to convince ourselves that it isn't harming anyone. We're really happy for them, aren't we?

But how happy do we feel after clicking out of social media? Do we truly feel a sense of happiness for them or do we feel a sense of dissatisfaction for our own lives? Do we walk away from the computer grateful for what we have or bitter for what we don't? Do we look at our homes and our families through eyes of joy or with one eye toward what someone else has?

Is it possible to use Facebook as a tool to stay connected in a busy world without allowing it to use us and bring on emotional upheaval? I believe it is. Here are a few reminders to help you avoid the emotional pit that Facebook and other social media can become.

1. **Remember it's the highlight reel!** Don't allow your brain to fill in the blanks from the small snippets of someone else's life that happens to appear on social media at any point in time. Think of your last vacation. Was every single second post-worthy? No, and neither was theirs.

2. **Remember what Theodore Roosevelt** said, "Comparison is the thief of joy." Refrain from making comparisons between your everyday life and your friend's highlight reel.

3. **Remember that others may feel the same about your posts at times**. It is often true that we want what we don't have. So even if your posts seem dull and uneventful, there are people who would see that as a wonderful and peaceful respite from their busy, chaotic lives.

4. **Remember to live your own life to the fullest**. Don't miss out by trying to Xerox life. *"Be yourself. An original is always worth more than a copy."*

Nutritional Health

Xenoestrogens

Xenoestrogens are endocrine disruptors that have estrogen-like effects.

Endocrine disruptors are a category of chemicals that alter the normal function of hormones. When our endocrine system releases hormones, those hormones send information to different tissues telling them what to do. When we are exposed to chemicals from the outside, the chemicals can mimic our natural hormones and block or bind hormone receptors. This causes a whole cascade of faulty programming, often resulting in disease states.

Estrogen is a natural hormone in humans that is important for things such as bone growth, healthy cholesterol levels, brain health, blood clotting and reproduction in men and women. The body regulates the amount needed through intricate biochemical pathways.

When xenoestrogens enter the body, they increase the total amount of estrogen resulting in a phenomenon called, estrogen dominance. Xenoestrogens are not biodegradable and are therefore stored in our fat cells. The build-up of xenoestrogens have been indicted in many conditions including breast, prostate and testicular cancer, obesity, infertility, endometriosis, early onset puberty, miscarriages and diabetes.

Limiting your exposure to xenoestrogens is immensely important for good health. Here is a list of things that are considered xenoestrogens. There is no way to create an exhaustive list but hopefully you can at least take steps to limit the ones listed. Some of these were also listed in Chapters F and M.

Skincare:
- **4-Methylbenzylidene camphor** (4-MBC)
- **Benzophenone**
- **Parabens** (anything with the word in it—usually at the end)
- **Stearalkonium Chloride**

Industrial Products and Plastics:
- **Bisphenol A** (monomer for polycarbonate plastic and epoxy resin; antioxidant in plasticizers)
- **DEHP** (plasticizer for PVC)
- **Phthalates** (plasticizers)
- **Polybrominated biphenyl ethers (PBDEs)** (flame retardants used in plastics, foams, building materials, electronics, furnishings, motor vehicles)
- **Polychlorinated biphenyls (PCBs)**

Food:
- **Butylated hydroxyanisole** / BHA (food preservative)
- **Erythrosine** / FD&C Red No. 3
- **Phenosulfothiazine** (a red dye)

Building supplies:
- **Pentachlorophenol** (general biocide and wood preservative)
- **Polychlorinated biphenyls / PCBs** (in electrical oils, lubricants, adhesives, paints)

Insecticides:
- **Atrazine** (weed killer)
- **DDT** (insecticide, banned)
- **Dichlorodiphenyldichloroethylene** (one of the breakdown products of DDT)
- **Dieldrin** (insecticide)
- **Endosulfan** (insecticide)
- **Fenthion**
- **Heptachlor** (insecticide)
- **Lindane / hexachlorocyclohexane** (insecticide, used to treat lice and scabies)

- **Methoxychlor** (insecticide)
- **Nonylphenol and derivatives** (industrial surfactants; emulsifiers for emulsion polymerization; laboratory detergents; pesticides)

Other:
- **Propyl gallate**
- **Chlorine and chlorine by-products**
- **Ethinylestradiol** (combined oral contraceptive pill)
- **Metalloestrogens** (a class of inorganic xenoestrogens)
- **Alkylphenol** (surfactant used in cleaning detergents

Here are a few practical guidelines to help you limit your exposure to xenoestrogens:
- Avoid pesticides, herbicides, and fungicides by choosing organic, locally-grown and in-season foods.
- Peel nonorganic fruits and vegetables. But remember that the chemicals get into the soil, thus getting into the root and into the food.
- Buy hormone-free meats and dairy products to avoid hormones and pesticides from the feed used.
- Reduce the use of plastics whenever possible.
  - o Storing food
  - o Covering food
  - o Plastic wraps
  - o Plastic water bottles
    Don't use them if you have a choice
    Never reuse them
    Never leave them in the sun
    If they have gotten hot, throw them out
    Never freeze them to drink later
- If you must microwave, never microwave food in plastic containers.
- Use glass or ceramics whenever possible to store food.
- Use chemical free, biodegradable laundry and household cleaning products.
- Choose chlorine-free products and unbleached paper products, such as tampons, menstrual pads, toilet paper, paper towels, and coffee filters.
- Use a chlorine filter on shower heads
- Filter drinking water
- Avoid creams and cosmetics that have toxic chemicals and estrogenic ingredients such as parabens and stearalkonium chloride.
- Minimize your exposure to nail polish and nail polish removers.

- Use naturally based fragrances, such as essential oils.
- Use chemical-free soaps and toothpastes.
- Read the labels on condoms and diaphragm gels.
- Be aware of noxious gas from copiers, printers, receipts, carpets, fiberboards, and at the gas pump.

Physical Health

X–traordinary Health

Throughout this journey you have learned many techniques that if followed lead to extraordinary health. Take some time to review your Physical Health notes. Has proper movement become a habit for you? Have you worked to perfect your form and move all joints in full ranges of motion? Are you using Active Release Techniques and Self Myofascial Release? Are you getting enough quality sleep and are you allowing yourself to recover well? Are you flossing your teeth and scraping your tongue? Is laughter a normal part of your life? Have you cleaned up your skincare/makeup to limit your chemical exposure? Have you found holistic ways to deal with pain, including foam rolling and correctives?

As you review your Physical Health notes, record below the areas that you have mastered and have become habit and celebrate! Then record the areas that you will commit to working on again. Give yourself a time-line.

I have mastered:

_____

_____

_____

_____

_____

I will continue to work on:

_____

_____

_____

_____

Cognitive Health

Xylophone

A xylophone, meaning "wooden sound" is a musical instrument in the percussion family that consists of wooden bars struck by mallets.

It will also score you a minimum of 24 points in Scrabble!

This week commit to playing a good old-fashioned game of Scrabble with your family or friends. It's fun, creates a bonding experience, fosters healthy competition, and is great exercise for your brain!

If you can't find the time for the old-fashioned way, check out Words with Friends on your computer or phone.

CHAPTER Y PREP

1. Begin Chapter Y's affirmation.
   Today, I say "YES, And!"
2. Foam roll daily and before workouts. Do only the corrective exercises that are still difficult for you. After foam rolling, use a dynamic warmup before beginning your workout.
3. Set appropriate and healthy boundaries and stick to them.
4. Continue to experiment with all six tastes.
5. Remain unmasked.
6. Take only the vitamins you know your body needs.
7. Use Brain Wave Vibration when you feel you need a "time-out."
8. Find the strengths behind your weaknesses.
9. Remember to live YOUR life, not someone else's.

CHAPTER Y

Emotional Health

Yes, And!

One of the things I absolutely love to watch is live improv! It amazes me how these comedians can receive anything and everything from another cast member and not only receive it but expand on it, bringing something new, and often hilarious, to the basic idea.

Shooting down someone's initial idea, even if you think it would be a horrible mistake, squashes creativity and imparts a sense of fear not only in the idea's originator but also in everyone around.

Try to take some time to watch improv videos on YouTube. It will make you laugh and will help you see the technique used.

This week, practice living a "yes, and" life. Whenever you can, gather the courage to say, "yes." It may lead you down a new path. Best of all, it will encourage creativity, boldness, freedom, and excitement in your own life and in the lives of those around you.

Nutritional Health

Your Personalized Nutrition Plan

Over the past several weeks you have experimented with foods and improved your nutrient content. You received a simple reminder of how to shop for your food—FOOD©—Free of anti-nutrients, Organic when possible, Original in form, Dense in nutrients.

Look back and record here the foods that have worked the best for you. What foods and supplements have increased your energy? Cleared your skin? Made your bowel movements more regular? Made you a nicer person to be around? Made your body composition more balanced? Focus on eating more of these, your very own superfoods.

My best breakfasts:

_____

_____

_____

_____

My best lunches:

_____

_____

_____

_____

My best dinners:

_____

_____

_____

_____

My best beverages:

_____

_____

_____

_____

My best snacks:

_____

_____

_____

_____

Physical Health

Yoga

Check out www.rhondahuff.com for the video lesson, "Chapter Y"

The word "yoga" translates to "yolk" or "to join." This is interpreted many different ways in the yoga community, but the most common interpretation is the joining and balancing between body, mind, and spirit. In the physical yoga practice, it refers to joining the breath with the physical postures or *asanas* (AH-sanas).

There are hundreds of benefits that yoga practitioners enjoy. These are just a few of them.

1.   Improves flexibility
2.   Builds muscle strength
3.   Improves posture
4.   Builds bone
5.   Increases blood flow
6.   Boosts immunity
7.   Lowers blood pressure
8.   Calms the mind
9.   Improves balances
10. Improves focus
11. Relieves tension
12. Aids sleep

In Vinyasa style yoga (also commonly known as "flow yoga"); the Sun Salutation or *Surya Namaskara* is the foundation of all flow. Our practice today will teach a basic Sun Salutation and demonstrate how it serves as the backbone for all different types of creative flows. There are a few slight variations of Sun Salutation, but most of the postures through the flow are the same. The video will take you through a Sun Salutation.

Here are the basic poses:

Tadasana (Mountain Pose)
Urdhva Hastasana (Upward Salute)
Uttanasana (Standing Forward Bend)
Ardha Uttanasana (Half Standing Forward Bend)
Chaturanga Dandasana (Four-Limbed Staff Pose)
Urdhva Mukha Svanasana (Upward Facing Dog)
Adho Mukha Svanasana (Downward Facing Dog)
Ardha Uttanasana (Half Standing Forward Bend)
Uttanasana (Standing Forward Bend)
Urdhva Hastasana (Upward Salute)
Tadasana (Mountain Pose)

The three main practices of yoga are meditation, breath practice or *pranayama,* and the physical practice that incorporates *asanas*. When regularly practiced together, yogis experience a balancing union of body, mind, and spirit.

Cognitive Health

Yawning

Did reading the title of this module make you spontaneously yawn? We have all heard that yawning is contagious. We yawn when we see someone yawn, hear someone yawn, and even when we see the word, "yawn." So how many times did you just yawn?

And though we yawn when we are tired, sleepy, waking up, and bored, there is another reason we yawn—to cool our brains. That's right! In the journal, *Medical Hypotheses*, Andrew Gallup of Princeton University and Gary Hack of the University of Maryland say that yawning helps regulate the brain's temperature. The go on to say, "The brain is exquisitely sensitive to temperature changes and therefore must be protected from overheating. Brains, like computers, operate best when they are cool."

The human maxillary sinus apparently flex during yawning like a bellows, which in turn cools the brain. In one study by Gallup, thermo-coupled probes were implanted in the frontal cortex of rats to measure brain temperature before, during, and after yawning. He reported that brain temperatures increased rapidly prior to yawning and decreased immediately after.

Another theory by Neuroscientist Andrew Newberg, M.D., and therapist Mark Robert Waldman, state that yawning is effective in reducing anger, stress, and anxiety, while enhancing awareness, calmness, alertness, and bodily relaxation. They suggest doing twelve to fifteen yawns with a few seconds between each one, taking two minutes to complete.

This discovery may be due to the cooling effect yawning has on the brain. This week try yawning. If you feel anxious or angry, take a two-minute timeout and yawn.

CHAPTER Z PREP

1. Take a few moments to get quiet. As you prepare for Chapter Z you should be relaxed and in a truly authentic, bold, and centered state of mind.

2. Repeat Chapter Z's affirmation as you quiet your mind
"I am ready to zero in. I am ready to live my best life."

3. Here are the affirmations that we used throughout the program. Slowly read through each affirmation, securing it in your mind and heart.
I fully love and accept myself just as I am right now.
Every part of my body is energized when I breathe.
I am open to positive change in all areas of my life.
I choose to stay calm in moments of stress.
I am a person of great worth.
I speak with integrity and ask for what I need.
I am grateful and blessed.
I am becoming the best version of myself.
I am making room in my life for what is ideal.
I am healthy in mind and body.
I am learning to be kind to others and myself.
I am learning to speak the love languages of others.
My mind is nourished and healthy.
I choose to see the positive things around me.
I am bold enough to own up to my mistakes.

I am at peace.

I look for the quality of interactions in my life.

I choose to respond, not react, to situations.

I set and respect healthy boundaries.

I am free to receive happiness in my life.

I am taking control of my health.

My heart and lungs are getting healthier every single day.

I have the power to turn my weaknesses into strengths.

I choose to live my life, not a Xerox copy of someone else's.

Today, I say "YES, and!"

Take a few moments to close your eyes, focus on a relaxing breath, and allow these truths to become a real part of you.

As you open your eyes, write your very own personal affirmation statement below.

My personal affirmation statement:

_____

_____

_____

_____

_____

CHAPTER Z

Check out www.rhondahuff.com for the video lesson, "Chapter Z"

Congratulations on making it to the last module! It is time to take what you have learned and really Zero-in on what is most important to you.

Please answer each question and carry the results forward to the appropriate chart.

Emotional Health

Have you learned to love and accept yourself just as you are right now?

Have you accepted that the path you are on is a marathon, not a sprint?

Have you realized that you are worthy of a wonderfully fulfilling and happy life?

Do you use your breath to relax, fall asleep, calm down?

Have you improved your life in the areas of:

Relationships?

Career?

Spirituality?

Physical activity?

Are you able to discern the difference between eustress (good stress) and distress (bad stress) and take actions to deal with any distress properly?

Are you remembering the Four Agreements?

Be impeccable with your word.

233

Don't take anything personally.

Don't make assumptions.

Always do your best.

Do you understand the purpose of grief, and have you been able to say goodbye to the things over which you have no control?

If you are a highly sensitive person, are you able to recognize instances that you may be over-reacting or taking things too personally and redirect your emotions?

Have you used your "ideal" list to help you keep your standards where you want them?

Has journaling helped you organize and understand your thoughts and feelings?

Do you take opportunities to perform random acts of kindness?

Do you allow your knowledge of love languages help you communicate and show love to those close to you?

Has knowing your inherent personality traits (Myers-Briggs) helped you better understand yourself and how you respond to the world around you?

Have you worked to work through negativity and to find more positives in your life?

Do you own up to your mistakes and also to your greatness?

Have you discovered peace in your day-to-day life?

Are you planning your schedule to have regular quiet time?

Are you able to respond instead of to react?

Have you set proper boundaries around the things that are important to you?

> Your time?
>
> Your energy?
>
> Your money?
>
> Your family?
>
> Other?

Are you successfully living an unmasked life?

Have you found the song within you?

Are you looking for the potential strengths in your weaknesses?

Are you living your own authentic life, without desiring a Xeroxed life of someone else?

Are you receiving what life throws at you with a resilient, "yes, and" attitude?

Please complete the following chart, noting areas that have been mastered and areas that you would like to continue to work on.

Emotional Health Successes	Emotional Health Continuations

Nutritional Health

What foods make you feel the best?

What foods have you eliminated or reduced?

Are you able to fast for twelve hours between dinner and breakfast?

Have you successfully spaced your meals four to five hours apart?

Do you have more energy?

Have your learned how to deal with cravings when they crop up and what triggers cravings in your life?

Are you following **FOOD**©?

Free of anti-nutrients (unpronounceables)

Organic when possible

Original in form

Dense in nutrients

Are you doing things to keep your gut healthy, such as eating fermented foods and taking probiotics?

Have you maintained a tidy and healthy kitchen?

Are you filling your plate with a rainbow of veggies and fruit?

Are you adding all six tastes into your nutrition plan? Sweet, salty, bitter, pungent, sour, astringent

Have you determined how much water per day is best for you?

Have you become more aware of the chemicals in our environment and food supply and taken steps to eat foods and use products that are whole, pure, and clean?

Please complete the following chart, noting areas that have been mastered and areas that you would like to continue to work on.

Nutritional Health Successes	Nutritional Health Continuations

Physical Health

Have you continued to use Self-Myofascial Release (foam rolling) to keep good circulation to the muscles and trigger points at bay?

Are you getting seven to nine hours of sleep per night with about three hours of deep sleep?

Are you in bed most days around 10 p.m. to maximize liver recovery (10 p.m.-2 a.m.)?

Has your posture been corrected?

Do your joints move in healthy, pain-free ranges of motion?

Are you laughing often?

Have you set up your exercise plan to include the following:

Foam rolling?

Corrective work?

Activities good for your dosha?

Exercises for each body part?

Horizontal PUSH (ex. Push up, Chest Press, Skullcrushers)

Horizontal PULL (ex. Rows of any kind)

Vertical PUSH (ex. Overhead Press, Push Press)

Vertical PULL (ex. Lat Pulldown, Pullups, Bicep Curls)

KNEE Dominant (ex. Squats, Lunges)

HIP Dominant (ex. Deadlift, Glute bridges)

Core

Metabolic

Rep ranges to meet your goal?

Goal	Rep goal for 1st set	Total Reps	Rest between sets
Strength	4-6	25	3 minutes
Hypertrophy (muscle size)	8-12	40	2 minutes
Endurance	15-20	60	less than 1 minute

Full-body movements that maximize your time and results?

A variety of movements that progresses as things get easier?

Training for the cardiovascular system?

Stretching?

Proper rest and recovery?
Yoga?

Please complete the following chart, noting areas that have been mastered and areas that you would like to continue to work on.

Physical Health Successes	Physical Health Continuations

Cognitive Health
What have you mastered?
ABC...ZYX?
Crosswords?
Dance?
Gratitude?

Self-hypnosis?
Improved intuition?
Juggling?
Map drawing?
Nondominance exercises?
Poetry?
Sudoku?
Brain teasers?
Vibration exercise?
Learning something new as a habit?
Scrabble?

Please complete the following chart, noting areas that have been mastered and areas that you would like to continue to work on.

Brain Health Successes	Brain Health Continuations

"The only person you are destined to become is the person you decide to be."
—Ralph Waldo Emerson

CELEBRATE THE NEW HEALTHIER YOU

Check out www.rhondahuff.com for the video lesson, "Celebrate"

Whew, what a journey! I am so proud of you! Give yourself a big pat on the back and a warm self-hug. You committed to improving your health by working hard through the program and you did it!

As we close out our time together, let's take a walk back to the Chapter A Prep. We covered three precepts to help you with your journey.

First, Be Authentic With Your Journey
Healing takes place where truth resides.

Second, Be Bold Enough to Stop Hiding From Yourself
Your life's purpose requires you, not a poor copy of someone else.

Third, Find Your Center
A mind at peace is stronger than the forces around you.

Can you remember your first thoughts and feelings around those three precepts? How do they differ today? And how do you move forward? Let me encourage you to continue the journey to health that you have begun. Review your notes anytime you need a refresher or a simple reminder.

Allow each new day to bring you gratitude, love, growth, and laughter. Take time to care for yourself so you can better serve others. Stay curious about your emotions and your experiences so you can continue to grow. Embrace change and challenge so you can share the wisdom learned with those coming behind you. May the truth of *authenticity*, the *boldness* of purpose, and the peace of being *centered* lead you on a path of indescribable joy.

And until we meet again, my friends… *JOURNEY ON.*

ABOUT THE AUTHOR

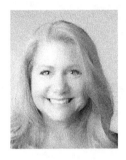

Rhonda Huff, CPT, CHHC, NLPH, AADP, is a subject matter expert in the fields of nutrition, fitness, and wellness. She has a BS in Fitness/Wellness with a concentration in rehabilitation and an M.Ed with a concentration in research and curriculum design. Rhonda is also a board-certified Holistic Health and Nutrition Coach through the Institute for Integrative Nutrition and the American Association of Drugless Practitioners, a certified Neuro-Linguistic and Hypnosis Practitioner through the NLP Center of New York, and is currently studying with the Institute for Functional Medicine. Rhonda is the owner of Glowing Swan Enterprises, LLC, the founder of Body-in-Balance Wellness & Fitness Studio, Rhonda Huff FIT, and the co-founder of the Center for Integrative Brain Health. Rhonda has helped thousands of people improve their lives through her online courses, speaking engagements, and private training services. Rhonda's last book, *The Addictive Personal Trainer: the client centered training approach that keeps them coming back for more*, was written to guide new personal trainers in how to establish themselves as experts in their field. Rhonda currently resides in Newport News, VA but also calls Boonville, NC and NYC home.

REFERENCES

Aron, Elaine. http://hsperson.com/test/highly-sensitive-test/

Bargh and Morsella. The Unconscious Mind. US National Library of Medicine. Perspectives on Psychological Science. 2008 Jan; 3(1): 73–79.doi: 10.1111/j.1745-6916.2008.00064.x

Bays HE. Safety considerations with omega-3 Fatty Acid therapy. American Journal of Cardiology. 2007;99(6A):S35-43.

Beck, J. S. (2011). Cognitive behavior therapy: Basics and beyond (2nd ed.). New York, NY: Guilford Press.

Berg, Dr. Eric. Understanding Body Types. www.drberg.com. Alexandria, VA.

Bowden, Jonny. The 150 Healthiest Foods on Earth. Gloucester, MA: Fair Winds Press, 2007.

Boyle, Mike. Advances in Functional Training. Aptos, CA: On Target Publications, 2010.

Brown, Brene. Rising Strong. New York, NY: Random House, 2015.

Buckley MS, Goff AD, Knapp WE, et al. Fish oil interaction with warfarin. Annals of Pharmacotherapy. 2004;38:50-2.

Chapman, Gary. The Five Love Languages, The Secret to Love that Lasts. Chicago, IL: Northfield Publishing, 2009.

Chopra, Deepak. Perfect Health. New York, NY: Three Rivers Press, 2000.

Cloud and Townsend. Boundaries. Grand Rapids, MI: Zondervan, 1992.

Cole GM. Omega-3 fatty acids and dementia. Prostaglandins Leukotrienes and Essential Fatty Acids. 2009;81(2-3):213-21.

Cook, Gray. Expanding on the Joint by Joint Approach. http://graycook.com/?p=35.

Cook, Gray. Movement: Functional Movement Systems: Screening, Assessment, Corrective Strategies. Aptos, CA: On Target Publications. 2010.

D'Adamo, Peter. Eat Right for Your Type. New York, NY: Penguin Putnam, 1996.

David, Marc. Mind over Food. The Institute for the Psychology of Eating.

Davies, Clair. The Trigger Point Therapy Workbook. Oakland, CA: New Harbinger Publications, 2004.

Dobson, K. S. (2012). Cognitive therapy. Washington, DC: APA Books.

Erasmus, Udo. Fats that Heal, Fats that Kill. Summertown, TN: Alive Books. 1993.

Gallup, Andrew. Yawning as a Brain Cooling Mechanism. http://academicminute.org/2014/10/andrew-gallup-suny-oneonta-yawns-are-cool/

http://adrenalfatiguesolution.com

http://ecoorganics.com

http://www.alz.org

http://www.alz.org/brain-health/brain_health_overview.asp

http://www.chronicpainresearch.org/Research

http://www.drweil.com/drw/u/QAA361058/what-is-leaky-gut.html#_ga=1.91319386.198319696
1.1461543453

http://www.eatingdisorders.org.au/eating-disorders/disordered-eating-a-dieting

http://www.ewg.org/skindeep/

http://www.messagebible.com

http://www.myersbriggs.org/my-mbti-personality-type/mbti-basics/c-g-jungs-theory.htm

http://www.t-nation.com

https://www.drugabuse.gov/publications/drugfacts/prescription-over-counter-medications

Institute for Functional Medicine. Immune Module, 2015. Hormone Module, 2016.

Institute for Integrative Nutrition Certification Program, 2012.

July 2006 - Volume 16 - Issue 4 - pp 283-292.

Lee, Ilchi. Brain Wave Vibration. Sedona, AZ: Best Life Media, 2009.

Magno and Kshirsagar. Ayurveda, A Quick Reference Guide. Lotus Press, Twin Lakes, WI, 2011.

Mercola, Joseph. How to Bring Minerals Back into the Soil and Food Supply. http://articles.
mercola.com/sites/articles/archive/2014/05/25/food-minerals-soil-health.aspx, 2014.

Nakayama, Andrea. Holistic Nutrition Lab Certification Program, 2013.

NLP Center of New York Certification Program, 2014.

Richards, Byron. Mastering Leptin. Minneapolis, MN: Wellness Resources, 2004.

Rogers, Sherry. The Cholesterol Hoax. Solvay, NY: Prestige Publishing, 2008.

Rosenthal, Joshua. Primary Foods. Institute for Integrative Nutrition. New York, NY.

Ruiz, Miguel. The Four Agreements. San Rafael, CA: Amber-Allen Publishing, 2012.

Russell, Jon, ed. The Journal of Musculoskeletal Pain. National Association of Myofascial Trigger
Point Therapists. Haworth Medical Press: Binghamton, NY,

Russell, Jon. The Fibromyalgia Syndrome. A Clinical Case Definition for Practitioners.
Binghamton, NY: Haworth Medical Press, 2003.

Selye, Hans. General Adaptation Syndrome, 1936.

Szabo, Sandor, Tache, Yvette, & Somogyi, Arpad. The legacy of Hans Selye and the origins of stress
research: A retrospective 75 years after his landmark brief "Letter" to the Editor of Nature.
Stress, September 2012; 15(5): 472–478.

Sheldon, Stevens, and Tucker. The Varieties of Human Physique, New York, NY: Harper, 1940.

Standard and Innovative Strategies in Cognitive Behavior Therapy - Edited by Dr. Irismar Reis De
Oliveira, 2012.

Starrett, Kelly. Becoming a Supple Leopard. USA: Victory Belt Publishing, 2013.

The Journal of Ayurveda and Integrative Medicine. Oct-Dec 2015.

The Myers Briggs Foundation, www.myersbriggs.org

Travis and Wallace, Dosha brain-types: A neural model of individual differences.

Updated Fluid Recommendation: Position Statement From the International Marathon Medical
Directors Association (IMMDA). Clinical Journal of Sport Medicine:

Wendt, Carsten. What is Deep Sleep and How Much do We Need? http://blog.addapp.io/deep-
sleep-much-need/

CPSIA information can be obtained
at www.ICGtesting.com
Printed in the USA
BVHW031604130819
555775BV00003B/294/P